Hepatitis A and Other Associated Hepatobiliary Diseases

Edited by Costin Teodor Streba, Cristin Constantin Vere, Ion Rogoveanu, Valeria Tripodi and Silvia Lucangioli

Published in London, United Kingdom

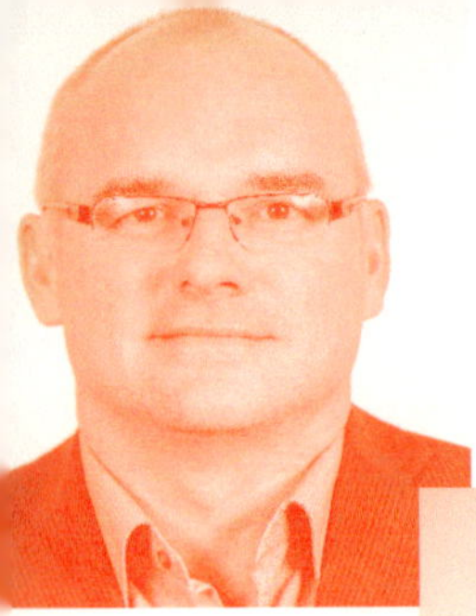
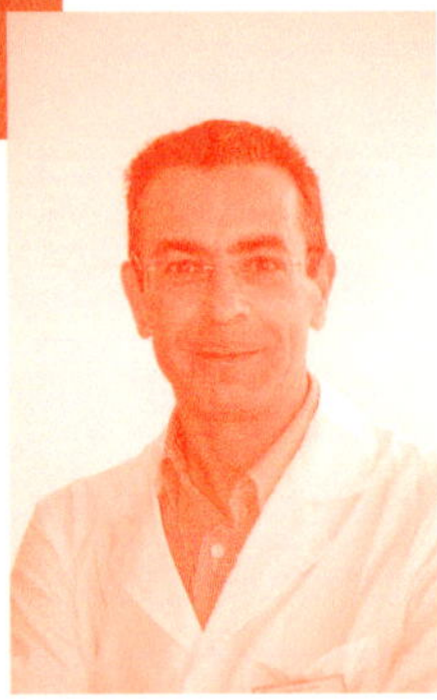
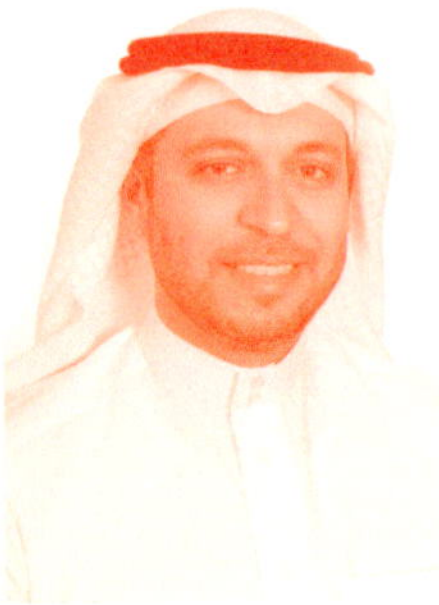
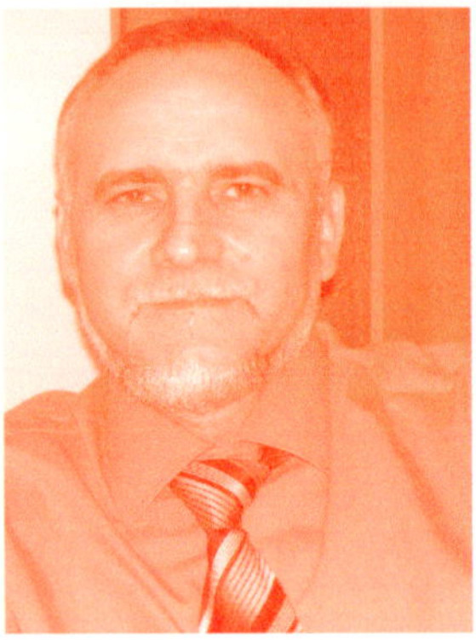
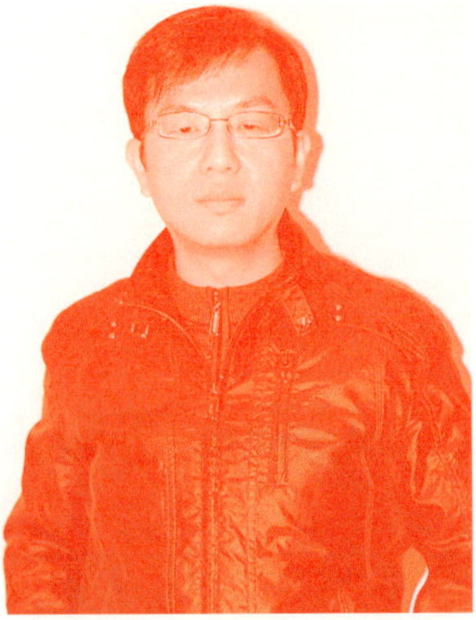
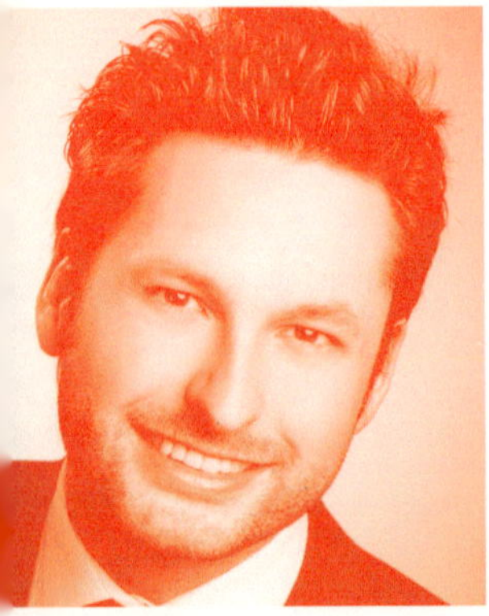
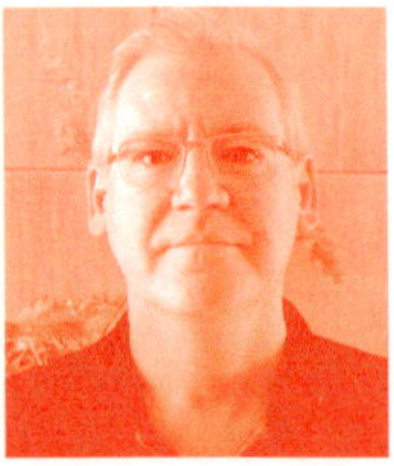

IntechOpen

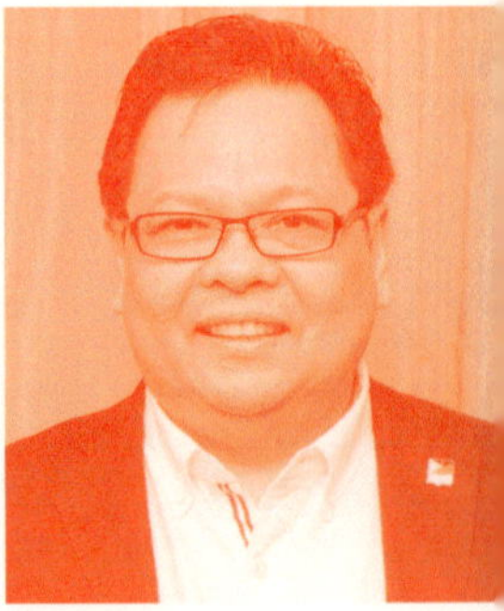
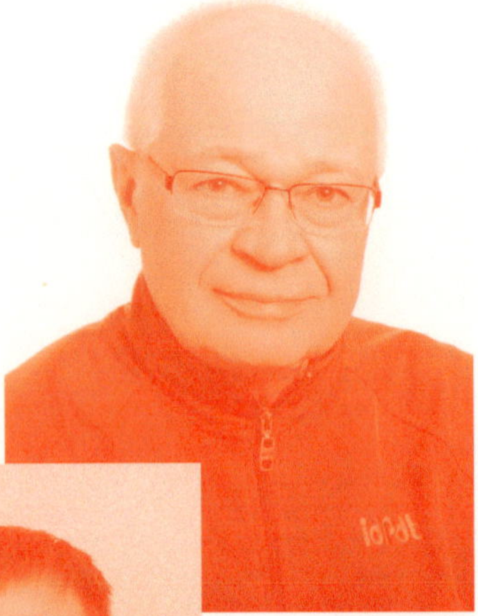
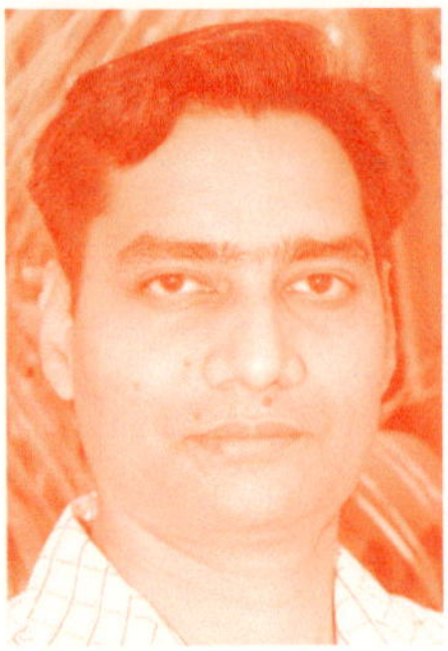
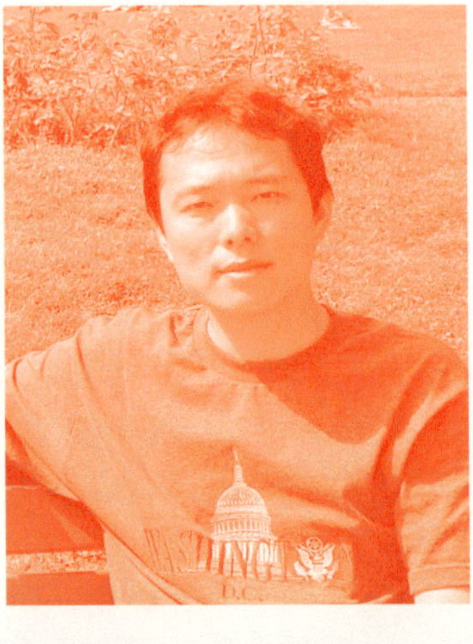
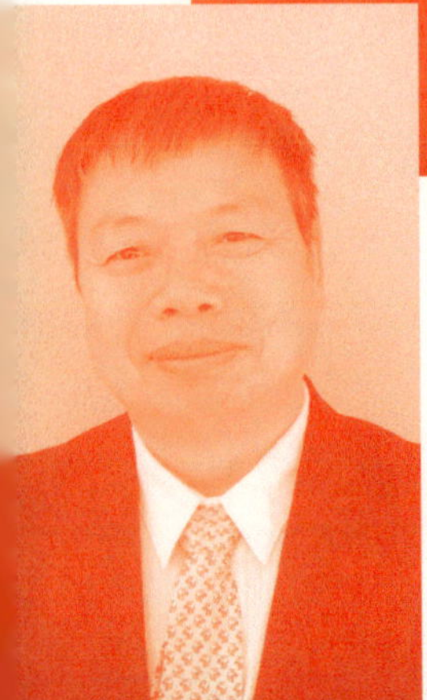
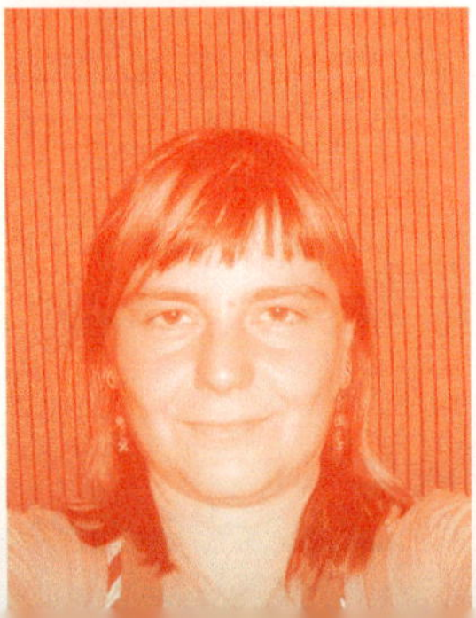

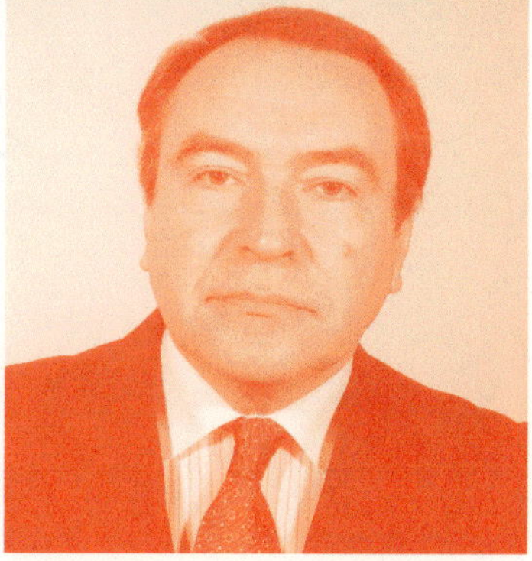
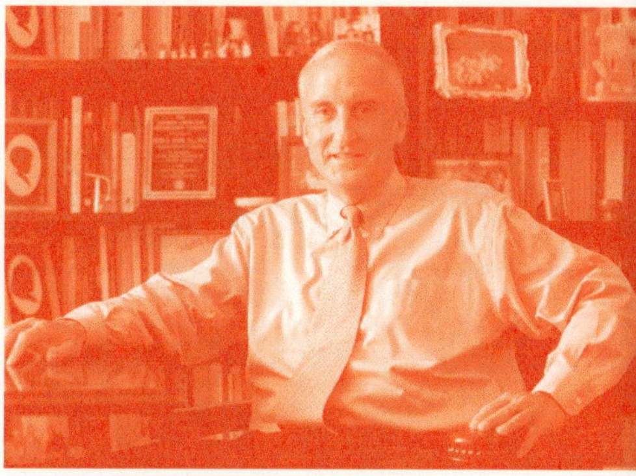
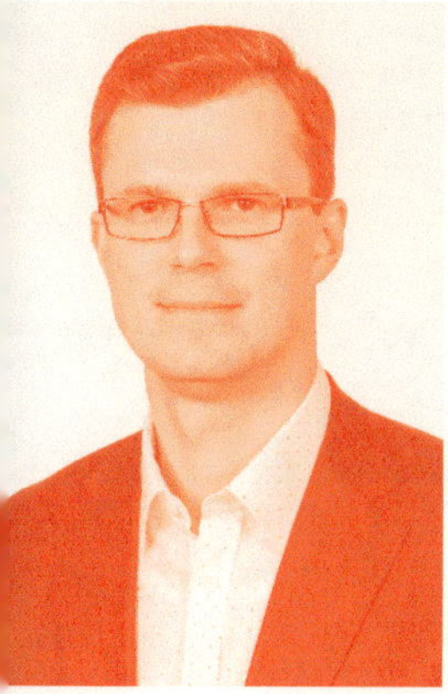
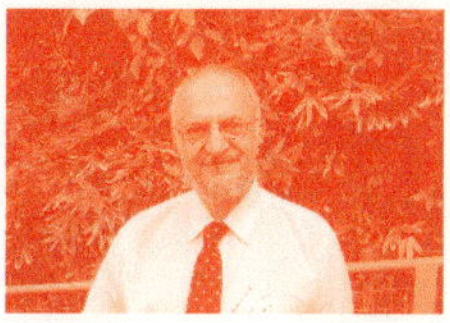
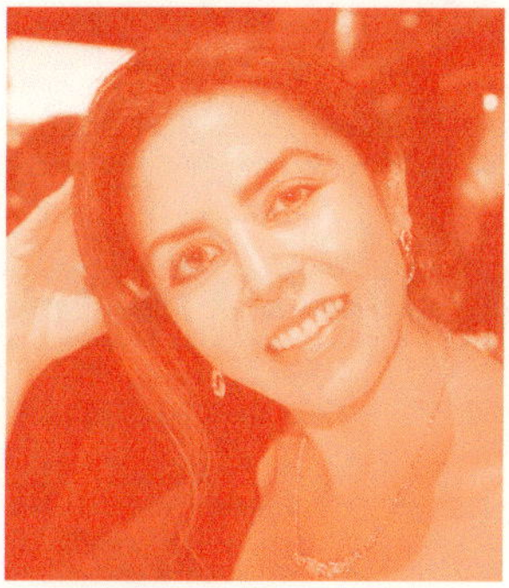

Supporting open minds since 2005

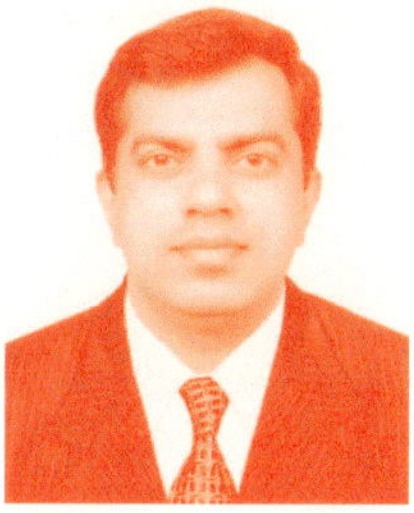
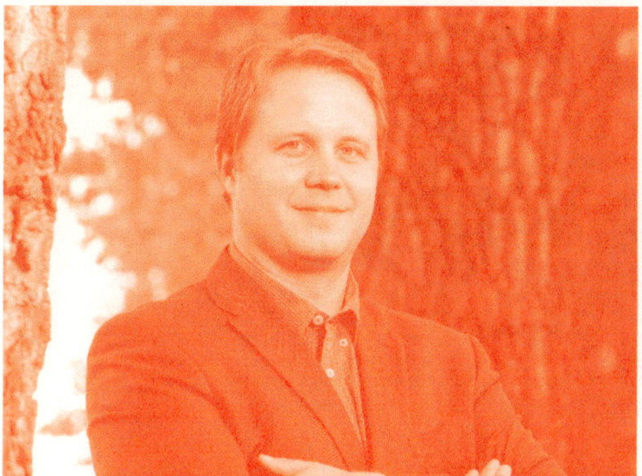
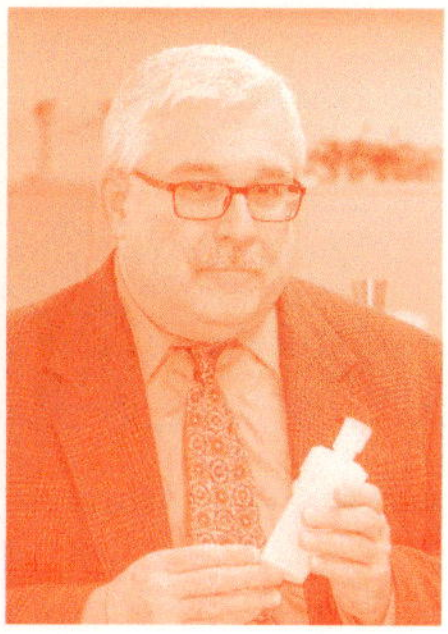
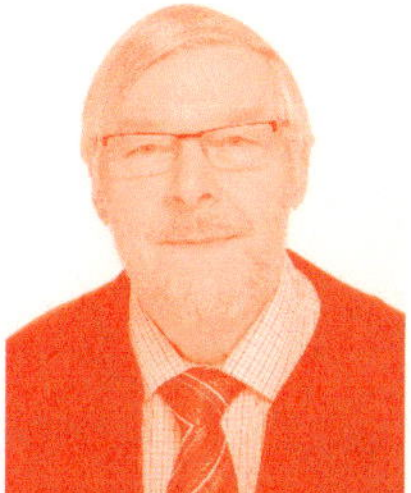
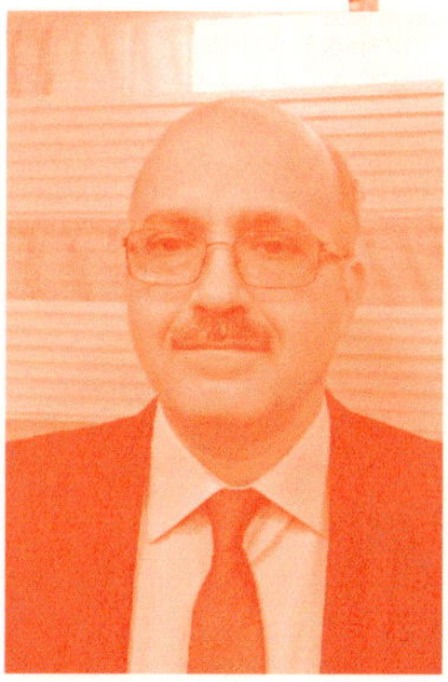
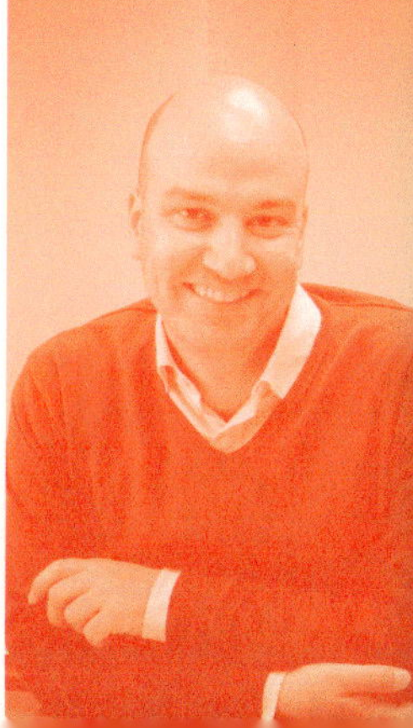
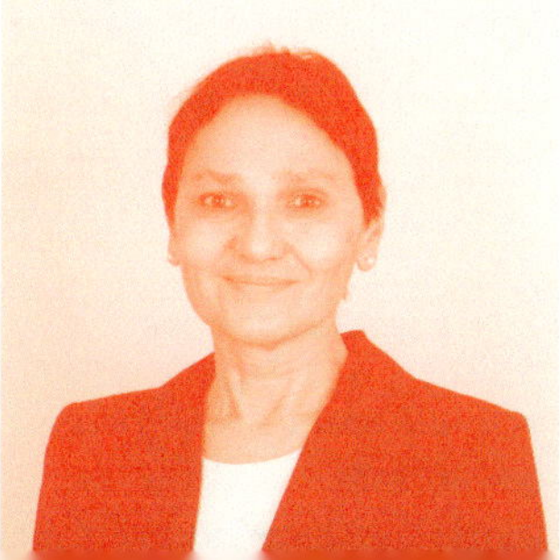

Hepatitis A and Other Associated Hepatobiliary Diseases
http://dx.doi.org/10.5772/intechopen.77707
Edited by Costin Teodor Streba, Cristin Constantin Vere, Ion Rogoveanu, Valeria Tripodi and Silvia Lucangioli

Contributors
Somanath Padhi, RajLaxmi Sarangi, Susama Patra, Subash Chandra Samal, Anita Chakravarti, Tanisha Bharara, Rosa Coelho, Guilherme Macedo, Valeria Tripodi, Silvia Lucangioli, Liliana Bianciotti, Manuela Martinefski, Adriana Rodrigues, Julia Teixeira Rodrigues, Priscila Liu, Saba Gargouri, Lamia Fki-Berrajah, Imen Ayadi, Amel Chtourou, Adnene Hammami, Héla Karray-Hakim, Huafeng Lin, Gang Li, Aiping Min, YanLei Chang, Lei Shi, Haizhen Wang, Sabina Wiecek, Damian Chukwu Odimegwu, Uzochukwu Gospel Ukachukwu

First published in London, United Kingdom, 2020 by IntechOpen
IntechOpen is the global imprint of INTECHOPEN LIMITED, registered in England and Wales, registration number: 11086078, 7th floor, 10 Lower Thames Street, London, EC3R 6AF, United Kingdom
Printed in Croatia

British Library Cataloguing-in-Publication Data
A catalogue record for this book is available from the British Library

Additional hard and PDF copies can be obtained from orders@intechopen.com

Hepatitis A and Other Associated Hepatobiliary Diseases
Edited by Costin Teodor Streba, Cristin Constantin Vere, Ion Rogoveanu, Valeria Tripodi and Silvia Lucangioli
p. cm.
Print ISBN 978-1-83880-672-9
Online ISBN 978-1-83880-673-6
eBook (PDF) ISBN 978-1-83880-674-3

For EU product safety concerns:
IN TECH d.o.o., Prolaz Marije Krucifikse Kozulić 3, 51000 Rijeka, Croatia, info@intechopen.com or visit our website at intechopen.com.

Meet the editors

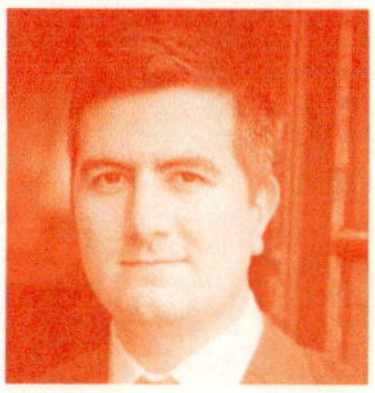

Streba Costin Teodor, MD, PhD, MSc, is Associate Professor at the University of Medicine and Pharmacy of Craiova and a member of the university's Research Center of Gastroenterology and Hepatology. His research focuses on diagnosis and histological image analysis in liver and pancreatic disease. Dr. Teodor specializes in devising medical-oriented diagnostic systems for gastrointestinal malignancies that integrate interpretation and computer-aided quantification of various imaging and clinical data. He has published many studies in various high-impact journals.

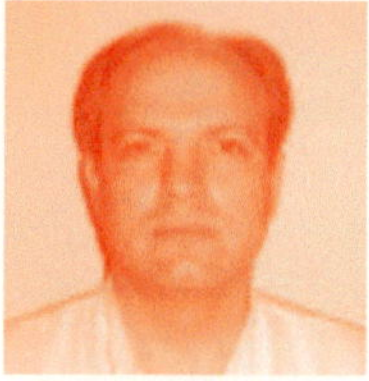

Vere Cristin Constantin, MD, PhD, MSc, is Professor of Gastroenterology at the University of Medicine and Pharmacy of Craiova and one of the founding members of the university's Research Center of Gastroenterology and Hepatology. His research interests span from neuroimmune mechanisms of gastrointestinal disease to novel diagnostic techniques in gastroenterology. Pioneering the introduction of wireless videocapsule in Romania, Dr. Constantin established a dynamic team of PhD and full-time scientists specialized in both medical sciences and bioinformatics. His publication record attests to his dedication for innovation in the field of gastroenterology and the complex integrative mechanisms that form the basis for this pathology.

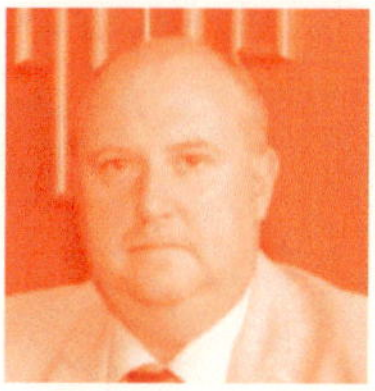

Rogoveanu Ion, MD, PhD, MSc, is Professor of Gastroenterology at the University of Medicine and Pharmacy of Craiova and one of the founding members of the university's Research Center of Gastroenterology and Hepatology. Mentoring a team of dedicated doctors and managing the curricular and scientific activities of the university as Rector, Dr. Ion is currently one of the lead authorities in ultrasound and power Doppler sonography, coordinating postgraduate courses for the past ten years. His most prestigious recent publications are all in the field of prevention, diagnosis, and treatment of hepatocellular carcinoma and various liver diseases.

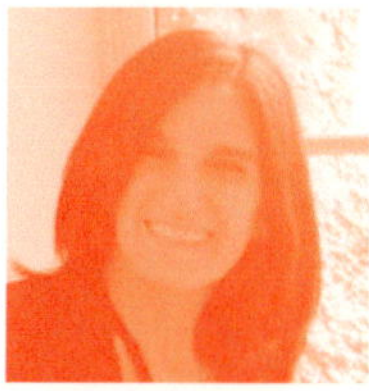

Prof. Dr. Valeria Tripodi is a biochemist with a master's degree and a doctorate in Molecular Biology and Genetic Engineering from the University of Buenos Aires (UBA). She is an Associate Professor in the Department of Pharmaceutical Technology, and Independent Researcher at the National Scientific and Technical Research Council (CONICET). She is the currently director of the Center for Pharmaceutical Development, Research and Control, in the Bioanalytics area. Prof. Tripodi has published more than sixty works in international journals, six book chapters, and four books. Since 1995, she has carried out extensive activity of technological transfer. Her main area of research focuses on the development of analytical methodologies applied to the diagnosis and monitoring of different pathologies. Currently, she is the coordinator of accreditation and self-evaluation and a senior advisor in the Faculty of Pharmacy and Biochemistry at UBA.

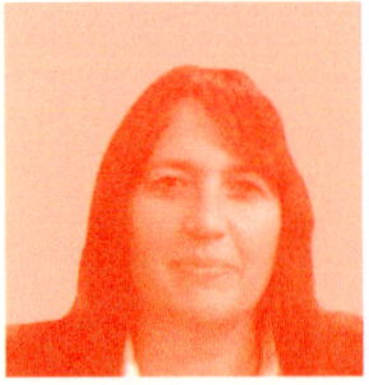

Dr. Silvia Lucangioli is Full Professor in the Pharmaceutical Technology Department at the Faculty of the Pharmacy and Biochemistry, University of Buenos Aires (UBA), and Investigator of the National Scientific and Technical Research Council (CONICET). She obtained a doctorate in Pharmacy, Biochemistry-Pharmaceutical Industries at the University of Buenos Aires. Her research focuses on the development of a miniaturized system for analytical methodologies and pharmaceutical formulations. Dr. Lucangioli has published more than eighty scientific articles, fifteen book chapters, and two books. She also supervises doctoral students. She is currently in charge of the Center of Research, Development and Pharmaceutical Control, Department of Pharmaceutical Technology (CIDEC), UBA, where is also Secretary for Technology Transfer.

Contents

Preface

Although the subject of acute viral hepatitis A may be exhausted, this book aims to prove otherwise. The addition of a selection of three of the most important topics in hepatobiliary diseases adds weight to the current scientific endeavors, making this volume even more appealing to the specialist community interested in the joint infectious and non-infectious pathologies of the liver.

With large-scale vaccination programs for hepatitis A, its global incidence has steadily decreased. However, it remains a threat in several areas of the world, and in the context of globalization and frequent travelling it may emerge as a reputable threat to some medical systems on the globe. This book begins by tackling interesting epidemiological aspects and debating implications for at-risk populations while placing the pathology in a historical context and exploring possible future trends.

The second part of the book examines animal models used in medical research of viral hepatitis A. It explores aspects of molecular biology and introduces the reader to fringe aspects such as the complex chemical interactions of natural products and mechanisms of viral infection. This section is anchored in current realities with an up-to-date report on the demographic shifts and paradigm changes that came with large-scale vaccination efforts.

Finally, the third section of the book presents novel insight into three of the most important biliary diseases: cholestasis, primary sclerosing cholangitis, and hemophagocytic lymphohistiocytosis.

This book will appeal to medical professionals in different areas of expertise as well as the broader medical community. We hope the information contained herein will spark interest and research in viral hepatitis A.

Streba Costin Teodor, MD, PhD, Msc, Vere Cristin Constantin, MD, PhD, Msc and Rogoveanu Ion, MD, PhD, Msc
University of Medicine and Pharmacy of Craiova,
Romania

Prof. Dr. Valeria Tripodi and Dr. Silvia Lucangioli
University of Buenos Aires,
Argentina

Section 1

Epidemiology of Hepatitis A

Chapter 1

Epidemiology of Hepatitis A: Past and Current Trends

Anita Chakravarti and Tanisha Bharara

Abstract

Hepatitis A virus is a common infectious etiology of acute hepatitis worldwide. It was not until World War II (1973) when hepatitis A virus was first identified by an American virologist, Stephen Mark Feinstone. The virus is most commonly transmitted through contaminated food, water, or sexual contact (oral-anal sex). The discovery of hepatitis A virus vaccine is considered a milestone in the history of acute viral hepatitis. Hepatitis A occurs worldwide and frequent outbreaks have been reported over the years. Major geographic differences have existed in endemicity of the disease depending primarily upon hygiene and sanitation practices. Some countries have experienced shifting of endemicity due to improvement of environmental hygiene, swelled International travel and national recommendations for hepatitis A vaccination. The age of acquiring hepatitis A virus is also shifting toward adolescents and adults. This has led to a more symptomatic disease, since hepatitis A infection among children is usually asymptomatic; this is known as the paradox of Hepatitis A epidemiology.

Keywords: acute hepatitis, vaccine, feco-oral route, men who have sex with men, outbreak, sero-prevalence, paradox of hepatitis A

1. Introduction

The discovery of hepatitis viruses is one of the most mesmerizing scientific escapades of the last five decades. Their identification has been considered a milestone that revolutionized modern day medicine [1]. Disease outbreaks resembling hepatitis A have been known since ancient times. The earliest accounts of contagious jaundice are traced to ancient China [2]. Feinstone et al. were first to identify Hepatitis A virus (HAV) in the year 1973 [3]. Increasing globalization poses fresh challenges for prevention of HAV infections. This chapter is an attempt to decipher the evolution of the disease over the years and summaries the current HAV situation around the world.

2. The breakthrough

Outbreaks resembling hepatitis A have been reported from Europe in the 17th and 18th centuries during the period of war. The pathologists Bamberger and Virchow proposed the name "catarrhal jaundice", as they believed the disease to be caused by mucus blockage of common bile duct [4]. Viral origin of the disease was first indicated by McDonald [5]. The virus was identified when the focus of

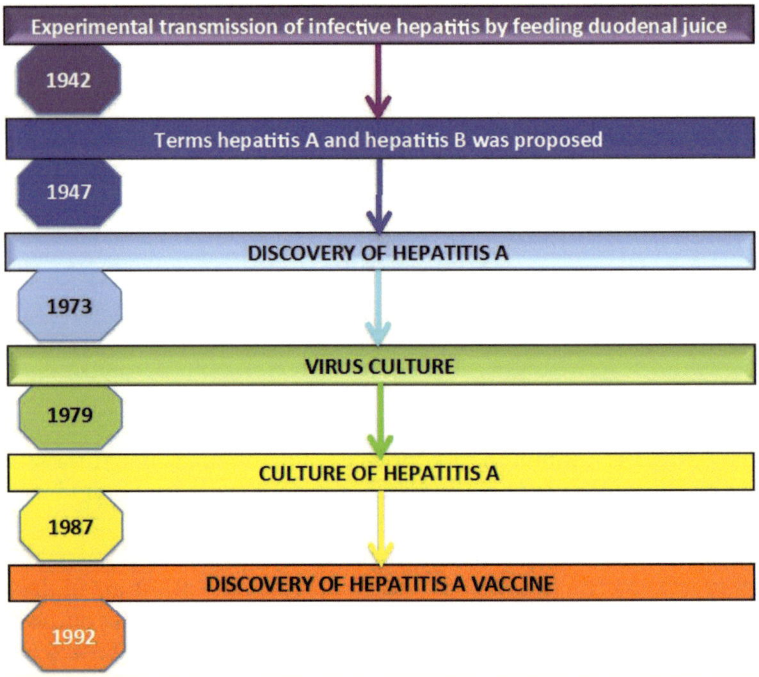

Figure 1.
The timeline of Hepatitis A virus.

investigation changed from serum to feces [6]. It was first seen under immune electron microscope in fecal suspension from infected Joliet prison inmates [3].

It was not until early 1900s that the mode of transmission of hepatitis A was identified [7, 8]. Although person-to-person contact was evident, the virus was thought to spread via droplet nuclei [9, 10]. Voegt successfully transmitted hepatitis A through duodenal juice. He published his findings in Munich Medical Weekly in 1942 [11]. Havens et al., at Yale University, United States of America, successfully transmitted jaundice by feeding serum and stool filtrate to 12 volunteers [12]. The differentiation between infectious hepatitis and serum jaundice was provided by a series of experiments carried out among mentally disabled residents at the Willowbrook State School, Staten Island [13]. While, it was MacCallum who proposed the terms hepatitis A and hepatitis B in the year 1947 [14]. The virus was first cultured in the year 1979 [15]. The viral genome was identified by reverse-transcriptase polymerase chain reaction. The cDNA copy was molecularly cloned. The RNA transcripts derived from cDNA clone proved infectious in cell cultures [16]. **Figure 1** depicts the timeline of Hepatitis A virus.

3. Hepatitis A virus – structure and mode of transmission

3.1 Structure

HAV is classified in the family Picornaviridae and genus Hepatovirus. HAV is a non-enveloped, 27- to 28-nm spherical virus with icosahedral symmetry. The virus contains a positive-sense, single stranded linear RNA. The 5′ end of the viral genome consists of a covalently bound protein termed VPg typical of picornaviridae. The viral genome consists of 60 copies each of its 3 major structural proteins, namely, VP1, VP2, and VP3 (1D, 1B, and 1C). Although a variety of genotypes (genogroups I–VII) have been identified by analysis of genome sequences, the virus has a single serotype. Individual strains of HAV have differences at the molecular level that may be useful for epidemiologic studies; however, a high degree of identity in nucleic acid (as high as 90%) and amino acid sequence (as high as 98%) is generally seen between strains [17, 18].

3.2 Mode of transmission

3.2.1 Feco-oral

HAV is a common infectious etiology of acute hepatitis worldwide. It is most commonly transmitted through the feco-oral route. Although, HAV contamination of food material can occur anytime during cultivation/preparation/distribution, it occurs most commonly during food distribution due to infectious food handlers [19]. Virtually any food may be contaminated with the virus. HAV is relatively resistant to extremes of temperature and pH. Hepatitis A virus is omnipresent; it can perpetuate on environmental surfaces, hands of food handlers, sewage as well as in a variety of food products [20].

3.2.2 Parenteral

Rare reports of transfusion related hepatitis A have been published over the years. Transmission is via blood/blood products (Factor VIII and IX) collected from an infected donor during the phase of viremia [21–23].

3.2.3 Sexual transmission

Studies have found that people who engage in sex with casual partners, sex in gay saunas, oral-anal intercourse and household or sexual contact with acute hepatitis A (AHA) patients are at increased risk of HAV infection. Several reports of HAV infections have been reported among men who have sex with men (MSM) [24–28].

4. HAV vaccine – the holy grail

The discovery of hepatitis A virus, its propagation in cell culture and cloning of its genome culminated almost two decades later in the development and licensing of an effective vaccine [29, 30]. According to the WHO, the most effective way to prevent HAV infection is to improve sanitation and immunization. Gamma globulin was found to be effective in prevention of measles in susceptible household contacts in the year 1944 [31]. Joseph Stokes, a pediatrician working at the University of Pennsylvania School of Medicine, used the knowledge in curtailing hepatitis A outbreak among children by administering gamma globulins [32].

First HAV vaccine was developed in early 1900 [33, 34]. In 1991, a preliminary study was published among vaccinees, demonstrating neutralizing antibodies following the administration of formalin-inactivated vaccines [35]. Live attenuated hepatitis A vaccine was developed subsequently [36].

By 1992, the clinical efficacy of two formalin-inactivated hepatitis A vaccines HAVRIX (Smith-Kline Beecham) and VAQTA (Merck, Sharpe and Dohme) became obvious [30, 33]. Two laboratory-attenuated strains HM175 and CR326F respectively were used for vaccine production. The adverse reactions following vaccination were minimal, and seroconversion after two doses was found to be quite high (99.8%) [30]. Other monovalent formalin inactivated HAV vaccines available in market today

Vaccine	Virus strain	Route of administration	Adjuvant	HAV antigen dose / injection Pediatric	Adult	Manufacturer
I. Formalin inactivated						
1. HAVRIX	HM-175	i.m	Aluminium hydroxide	720 ELU	1440 ELU	GlaxoSmithKline
2. VAQTA	CR-326	i.m	Aluminium hydroxide	25U	50U	Merck, Sharpe and Dohme
3. AVAXIM	GBM	i.m	Aluminium hydroxide	80U	160 U	Aventis Pasteur
4. HEALIVE	TZ84	i.m	Aluminium hydroxide	250 U	500U	Sinovac Biotech Co LTd
5.Weisairuian	Lv-8	i.m	Aluminium hydroxide	320 ELU	640 ELU	Institute of Medical Biology of the Chinese Academy of Medical Sciences; Kunming
6.Veraxim	YN5	i.m	Aluminium hydroxide	800 ELU	1600 ELU	Shanghai Wison Bioengineering Inc
7. EPAXAL	RG-SB	i.m	Virosomes	24U	24U	Crucell/ Berna Biotech
8. TWINRIX	HM-175	i.m	HM-175	-	1 ml (720 ELU HAV+ 20μg HBsAg)	GlaxoSmithKline
II. Live attenuated						
1. Freeze-dried live HAV vaccine	H2	s.c	None	0.5 ml	1ml	Zhejiang Pukang Biotech company
2. HAVAC Freeze-dried live HAV vaccine	LA-1	s.c	None	-	1ml	Changchun Institute of Biologic Products

Table 1.
List of HAV vaccines available in market.

include AVAXIM (Aventis Pasteur), HEALIVE (Sinovac Biotech Co Ltd), Weisairuian (Institute of Medical Biology of the Chinese Academy of Medical Sciences; Kunming), Veraxim (Shanghai Wison Bioengineering Inc) and EPAXAL (Crucell/Berna Biotech). Hepatitis A vaccine is also available as a combined preparation with Hepatitis B vaccine in the form of TWINRIX (GlaxoSmithKline) **Table 1** [37–39].

The Food and Drug Administration (FDA) licensed HAVRIX in February 1995 for children (≥2 years), adults and travelers [34]. Centers for Disease Control and Prevention recommends vaccination for children 12 months or older, travelers to endemic countries, gays, illegal drug users, individuals with occupational risk exposure and chronic liver disease patients. The American College of Physicians too also recommends vaccination of high-risk groups [40].

In the United States, vaccination against hepatitis A is available as inactivated, monovalent vaccines (HAVRIX and VAQTA) or in combination with hepatitis B (TWINRIX). These vaccines are highly efficacious with seroconversion rates approaching 100% [41]. With the implementation of vaccination, the incidence of HAV in the United States has shown a drastic decline of 92% (12 cases per 100,000 in 1995 to 1 case per 100,000 in 2007) [42].

Among the developing nations, Indian Academy of Pediatrics (IAP) recommends two doses of vaccine for children (≥1 year). The recommended dose is 720 ELISA Units (ELU) for <19 years and 1440 ELU for ≥19 years. Protective antibody titers are seen in almost 100% vaccinees following the second dose [43]. No major adverse reactions have been associated with vaccine use.

CDC recommends vaccine instead of immunoglobulin for exposure to HAV in healthy individuals aged 1 to 40 years. Standard adult dosing recommends administration of two doses of the vaccine 6–12 months apart. For individuals 41 years and older, immunoglobulin administration is preferred due to the risk of more severe clinical presentation and limited evidence of vaccine efficacy in this age group. Immunoglobulins are also recommended for children less than 12 months, individuals with chronic liver disease, and immunocompromised patients [44–46].

5. HAV epidemiology – pre-vaccine era and the paradox of vaccine era

5.1 The pre-vaccine era

In the pre-vaccine era, hepatitis A occurred in cycles, every 10–15 years, with majority of cases reported among children (≤15 years) [47, 48]. Most cases (12–25%) of hepatitis A in the United States occurred as communitywide epidemics in which infection was transmitted from person to person among household or sexual contacts. International travel and foodborne outbreaks accounted for a small percentage of cases [49]. Asymptomatic infections among children played an important role in sustaining transmission. According to a survey conducted in the United States of America (1988–1994), a third of the population were sero-positive for anti-HAV IgG antibodies [50]. In the developing part of the world, majority of the population acquires asymptomatic hepatitis A infection early in life, such that large proportion of population is immune to HAV [51, 52].

HAV infection resulted in devastating consequences in susceptible populations. An outbreak in Shanghai, China in 1988 affecting over 300,000 people due to consumption raw clams represents an example of the magnitude problem in the pre-vaccine era [53].

5.2 The vaccine era

5.2.1 The world scenario – HAV sero-prevalence

WHO estimates that approximately 1.5 million people are infected with HAV each year [54]. The incidence of HAV in a given population correlates with socioeconomic properties such as income, density of housing, sanitation, and water quality. Endemic rates are high in developing countries with poor sanitation and hygiene practices. HAV endemicity is classified into low, intermediate, and high based on the sero-prevalence of anti-HAV IgG (<15%, 15–50% and >50%) [37]. High sero-prevalence reflects that majority of the population is immune to HAV [55]. HAV in children is usually asymptomatic, while frank hepatitis is seen when HAV infection occurs in adults. Since 1999 several countries including, southern Asia, Latin America, and Europe, have experienced a decline in the incidence of HAV infection due to improved sanitation and routine vaccination. This has resulted in a higher incidence of HAV infection among adult population [56–61]. The shift in age group, which acquires hepatitis A, towards adolescents and adults has amplified the incidence of symptomatic disease, since childhood HAV infection is usually asymptomatic [51, 52].

Since the availability of HAV vaccine, an overall increase in the incidence of reported HAV cases has been observed from European Union countries [62]. This points to new risks associated with globalization and population migration [62, 63]. According to a health survey conducted in the USA, a significant decrease in HAV immunity among adult population was noted between 1988–1994 and 1999–2006 [64]. The survey also demonstrated rise in the rate of hospitalization among HAV infected individuals, consequent to a higher percentage of symptomatic infection among adult population over the last decade [65]. This is known as the "paradox of hepatitis A risk" [55].

Prognosis of HAV is usually good among younger population, with low mortality rates (0.1%). The mortality rate increases proportionately with age, to as high as 2.1% among ≥40 years old [66]. In developing world, including Asia, Africa and South America, evidence of past infection is nearly universal. Juxtapose to this, infection rates are low in developed countries such as the United States, Canada, and Europe. High-risk groups in these regions comprise of injection drug users, homosexuals, people traveling to endemic regions, and among isolated communities such as nursing homes etc. [67].

In the USA, HAV outbreaks were common among illicit drug users in the pre-vaccine era. Drug users accounted for over 20% of all HAV cases as reported by the CDC during mid-1980s [68, 69]. Since 1999, with the implementation of routine HAV vaccination program, hepatitis A incidence has shown a steady decline until 2011 [70, 71]. The incidence has stabilized at an annual average of over a 1000 cases per year. Most cases were reported among international travelers returning from countries endemic for HAV [72].

In a sero-prevalence study conducted among military personals in France, Lagarde found the prevalence of HAV antibodies as 16.3% [73]. Another study conducted in Korea found the overall HAV sero-prevalence of 63.8% [74]. Japan has been conducting sero-prevalence studies over the years. The overall HAV sero-prevalence has dramatically decreased from 96.9% in 1973 to 96.9% in 1984 and 12.2% in 2003. Notably, the population susceptibility increased annually [75]. A sero-prevalence survey in Taiwan during 2009–2010 showed that only 10% of MSM aged 18–40 years in Taiwan had anti-HAV antibodies [76]. HAV vaccination program was implemented in Taiwan in 2016. Although this lead to decline in the frequencies of both human cases and positive sewage samples, no substantial increase in vaccination coverage was seen among high risk groups like MSM and HIV-infected patients [77].

Exposure to HAV is virtually universal before the age of 10 years in most developing countries [78]. In a study conducted in rural Liberia, an annual incidence of HAV was reported to be 45% among children aged 1–5 years [79]. In Indonesia, 95% of children, under the age of 10 years, were naturally immune to HAV infection [80]. Above-mentioned studies point towards the fact that, mass HAV vaccination might not be necessary in highly endemic regions.

In India, the sero-prevalence of anti-HAV antibodies exceeds 90% among adults [81]. However, there have been recent reports of a decreasing sero-prevalence across the country, paralleling with the industrialized world [82, 83]. Accordingly, HAV vaccination has been recommended for school children as well as adults [84]. Another study conducted among children found the age-related sero-prevalence of HAV to be 50.3% in the age group of 6–10 years and 30.3% among 18 months to 6 years of age. The HAV prevalence correlated strongly with the child's education and socioeconomic status [85]. In another Indian study, the HAV prevalence was found to be 97.2% [78]. These findings were in agreement with the expected pattern of HAV sero-prevalence in an area of high endemicity. Similar findings have been reported from other parts of the country as well [86–88].

About 90% of Indian children acquire protective antibodies against HAV by the age of 10 years. Similar patterns of endemicity have been found in other developing countries, with high sero-prevalence of anti-HAV antibodies [89]. Surveys conducted among children in Egypt have also reported almost 100% sero-prevalence rates [90].

Several studies from India have recently reported a significant sero-epidemiological shift, with increasing incidence of infection among adults and adolescents. Recently in New Delhi, anti-HAV antibody prevalence among adults was reported to be as low as 36.7% [82].

Chile and Jordan have reported a decrease in anti-HAV sero-prevalence over the years [89, 91]. The study conducted in Jordan showed a continual rise of the sero-prevalence rates with rise in age. While, sero-prevalence was 26% among <2 years old, the rate increased to a whooping 94% for >20 years old [91]. A study conducted in Western Brazil revealed overall sero-prevalence among children as 16.7% in the year 2011, which significantly increased to 70.45% in a recently conducted survey [52, 91]. This high prevalence might be attributed to disease outbreaks in few parts of the district of Gampaha.

5.2.2 HAV outbreaks over the last decade

Over the last 10 years, several outbreaks have been reported throughout the world **Table 2** and **Figure 2** [92–107].

Although feco-oral route has been implicated in most of the cases, sexual mode of transmission among high risk groups is the second most prevalent route of transmission [104, 105].

In 2016, about 2000 cases of HAV were reported in the United State [92]. CDC and FDA investigated two major HAV outbreaks due to consumption of contaminated foods (strawberries imported from Egypt and scallops from Philippines). The first outbreak affected 134 people, with two hospitalization while, the second outbreak affected 292 individuals with 94 hospitalizations [93, 94]. An HAV outbreak in California in 2017 encompassed homelessness individuals and illicit drug users with poor sanitation practices. The outbreak spread to several other states as well. A total of 694 individuals were infected, with 45 hospitalizations and 21 deaths [95].

A sizeable hepatitis A outbreak was reported in Australia in 2009, resulting in a 2-fold increase in the number of cases reported to the state health departments. Surveillance data suggested infection due to contaminated semidried tomatoes [96].

S. No.	Year	Geographical Location	No. of documented cases	Route of transmission	Source of infection
1.	2009	Autralia	Not specified	Feco-oral	Semi-dried tomatoes
2.	2010	London	5	Feco-oral	-
3	2011	Korea	16	Feco-oral	-
2.	2013	India (Lucknow)	267	Feco-oral	-
3.	2014	India (Mylapore village)	45	Feco-oral	Contaminated water
4.	2015	Taiwan	Not specified	Sexual	MSM
5.	2016	USA (9 states)	134	Feco-oral	Strawberries
6.	2016	USA (Hawaii)	292	Feco-oral	Scallops
7.	2016	Europe	Not specified	Sexual	MSM
8.	2016	India (Kerala)	223	Feco-oral	Food from newly opened hotel
9.	2017	USA (California)	694	?Feco-oral	Illicit drug users/homeless
10.	2018	Europe	163	? Feco-oral	Travel

Table 2.
Hepatitis A outbreaks around the world over the last decade.

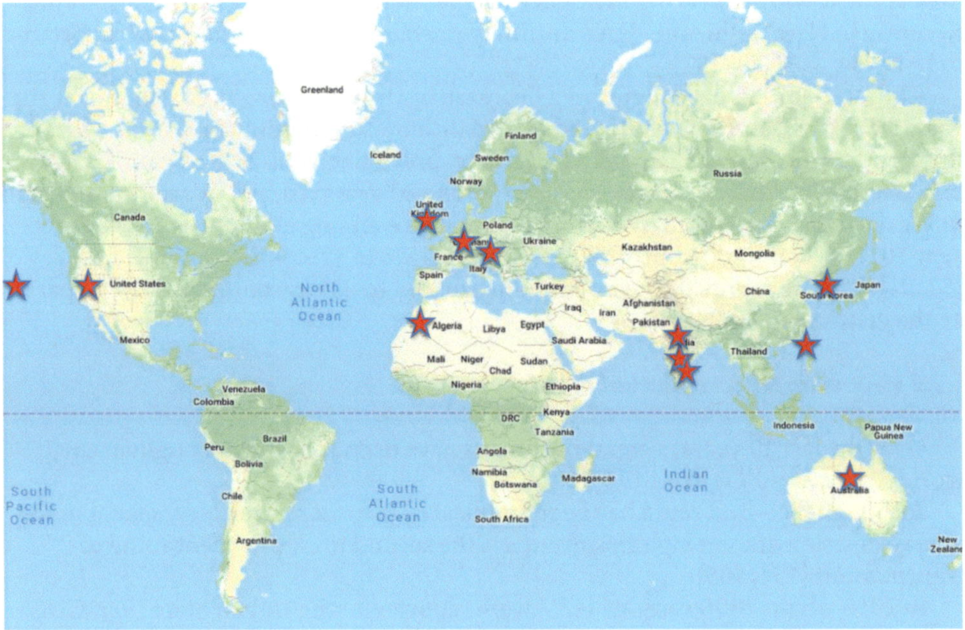

Figure 2.
Hepatitis A outbreaks throughout the world over the last decade.

A total of 32 outbreaks of water/food-borne disease outbreaks were reported from Kerala, India alone, in the same year, involving 2421 cases. All these outbreaks were attributable to feco-oral route [97]. Around 223 hepatitis A cases were identified in a HAV outbreak in Kerala. Attack rate was found to be highest among the age group of 16–30 years (1.44%). Food/water from a newly opened hotel in the area was the possible source of the outbreak [101]. In another study, authors reported

HAV outbreak in the medical college area in Kottayam [100]. Another outbreak of acute hepatitis was reported from Mylapore village, Kollam district, southern India during February to June 2013. A total of 45 cases were affected, pipe water contamination from a bore well was identified as the source [101].

In a study conducted among acute viral hepatitis patients in North India, hepatitis A virus was identified as the most common etiological agent (26.96%) followed by hepatitis E virus [99].

Gassowski et al. reported two hepatitis A outbreaks in Europe. One affecting travelers returning from Morocco and the other among European residents without travel history. The outbreaks lasted from January to June 2018, affecting 163 patients in eight European countries. The HAV was genotypically identified as belonging to subgenotype IA DK2018-231 and subgenotype IB V18–16428. Common risk factor among the cases was found to be unvaccinated travel due to lack of awareness [102].

In July 2010, five cases of HAV infection were reported among the Orthodox Jewish (OJ) community in London, United Kingdom. Two of the cases gave history of travel to Israel for the same event a few days back. A total of 900 contacts of the cases were traced and vaccinated [106].

Cyclic outbreaks of HAV among high-risk groups (MSM and/ HIV) have been described in several reports. Outbreak strains among MSM across countries were found to be genetically alike and circulated for over a decade [104, 105]. In June 2015, a considerable increase in reports of AHA infection was noted in Taiwan mostly affected MSM and patients with HIV or other STI. The strain was later identified as TA-15 strain. In 2016, multi-country HAV outbreaks predominately affecting MSM were observed in Europe. The EuroPride strain (RIVM-HAV16–090) detected was genetically quite similar to the TA-15 strain identified earlier [87, 108]. A similar outbreak strain was also reported in the United States in 2017 [103], which suggests a global pattern of increased risk among susceptible male adults, with possible transmission through sexual contacts at MSM events.

6. Conclusion

HAV adversely affects the economy of a country by decreasing productivity of its citizens due to absenteeism from work, adding to medical costs and the effect on tourism. Improving sanitary conditions and providing clean drinking water are imperative pillars in curtailing spread of HAV. Simple method like hand hygiene is an effective way to prevent virus transmission. Vaccination forms the foundation in prevention of HAV. Both inactivated and live attenuated vaccines are licensed and available for use. Improved sanitation and vaccination although prevents Hepatitis A infection, it paradoxically increases the susceptibility of adult population towards a more symptomatic disease. This vicious cycle is the dilemma of HAV control and prevention program.

Conflict of interest

The authors declare no conflict of interest.

Author details

Anita Chakravarti* and Tanisha Bharara
Department of Microbiology, Shree Gurugobind Singh Tricentenary University, Gurugram, Haryana, India

*Address all correspondence to: anitachakravarti@gmail.com

References

[1] Trepo C. A brief history of hepatitis milestones. Liver International. 2014;**34**:29-37

[2] Zuckerman AJ. The history of viral hepatitis from antiquity to the present. In: Deinhardt F, Deinhardt J, editors. Viral Hepatitis: Laboratory and Clinical Science. New York: Marcel Dekker; 1983. pp. 3-32

[3] Feinstone SM, Kapikian AZ, Purcell RH. Hepatitis A: Detection by immune electron microscopy of a virus like antigen associated with acute illness. Science. 1973;**182**:1026-1028

[4] Gruber W, Virchow R. Occurrence and diagnosis of the hepatic, and in particular, the catarrhal icterus. Virchows Archiv. 1865;**32**:117-125

[5] McDonald S. Acute yellow atrophy of the liver. Edinburgh Medical Journal. 1907;**1**:83

[6] Feinstone SM. History of the discovery of hepatitis A virus. Cold Spring Harbor Perspectives in Medicine. 2019;**9**(5):9-22

[7] Cockayne EA. Catarrhal jaundice, sporadic and epidemic, and its relation to acute yellow atrophy of the liver. QJM: An International Journal of Medicine. 1912;**6**:1-29

[8] Willcox WH. The epidemic jaundice of campaigns. British Medical Journal. 1916;**1**:297-300

[9] Blumer G. Infectious jaundice in the United States. JAMA. 1923;**81**:353-358

[10] Cullinan ER. The epidemiology of jaundice. Proceedings of the Royal Society of Medicine. 1939;**32**:933-950

[11] Voegt H. Zur aetiologie der hepatitis epidemica. Munchener medizinische Wochenschrift. 1942;**89**:76-79

[12] Havens WP, Ward R, Drill VA, Paul JR. Experimental production of hepatitis by feeding icterogenic materials. Proceedings of the Society for Experimental Biology and Medicine. 1944;**57**:206-208

[13] Krugman S, Ward R, Giles JP. The natural history of infectious hepatitis. The American Journal of Medicine. 1962;**32**:717-728

[14] Anonymous.Homologous serum hepatitis. Lancet. 1947;**ii**:691-692

[15] Provost PJ, Hilleman MR. Propagation of human hepatitis A virus in cell culture *in vitro*. Proceedings of the Society for Experimental Biology and Medicine. 1979;**160**:213-221

[16] Cohen JI, Ticehurst JR, Feinstone SM, Rosenblum B, Purcell RH. Hepatitis A virus cDNA and its RNA transcripts are infectious in cell culture. Journal of Virology. 1987;**61**:3035-3039

[17] Nainan OV, Xia G, Vaughan G. Diagnosis of hepatitis A virus infection: A molecular approach. Clinical Microbiology Reviews. 2006;**19**:63-79

[18] Lemon SM, Jansen RW, Brown EA. Genetic, antigenic and bio- logical differences between strains of hepatitis A virus. Vaccine. 1992;**10**(1):40-44

[19] Acheson D, Fiore AE. Hepatitis A transmitted by food. Clinical Infectious Diseases. 2004;**38**(5):705-715

[20] Sattar SA, Jason T, Bidawid S, Farber J. Foodborne spread of hepatitis A: Recent studies on virus survival, transfer and inactivation. Canadian Journal of Infectious Diseases. 2000;**11**:159-163

[21] Mannucci PM, Gdovin S, Gringeri A. Transmission of hepatitis A to patients with hemophilia by factor VIII concentrates treated with organic solvent and detergent to inactivate viruses. The Italian collaborative group. Annals of Internal Medicine. 1994;**120**:1-7

[22] Lemon SM. The natural history of hepatitis A: The potential for transmission by transfusion of blood or blood products. Vox Sanguinis. 1994;**67**(4):19-23

[23] Soucie JM, Robertson BH, Bell BP. Hepatitis A virus infections associated with clotting factor concentrate in the United States. Transfusion. 1998;**38**:573-579

[24] Henning KJ, Bell E, Braun J, Barker ND. A community-wide outbreak of hepatitis A: Risk factors for infection among homosexual and bisexual men. The American Journal of Medicine. 1995;**99**(2):132-136

[25] Kuijpers LA, Kool JL, Veugelers PJ, Coutinho RA, Griensven GJ. An outbreak of hepatitis A among homosexual men in Amsterdam, 1991- 1993. International Journal of Epidemiology. 1995;**24**(1):218-222

[26] Bell A, Ncube F, Hansell A, Davison KL, Young Y, Gilson R, et al. An outbreak of hepatitis A among young men associated with having sex in public venues. Communicable Disease and Public Health. 2001;**4**(3):163-170

[27] Beebeejaun K, Degala S, Balogun K, Simms I, Woodhall SC, Heinsbroek E, et al. Outbreak of hepatitis A associated with men who have sex with men (MSM), England, July 2016 to January 2017. Euro Surveillance. 2017;**22**(5):304-354

[28] Mazick A, Howitz M, Rex S, Jensen IP, Weis N, Katzenstein TL, et al. Hepatitis A outbreak among MSM linked to casual sex and gay saunas in Copenhagen, Denmark. Eurosurveillance. 2005;**10**(5):536

[29] Maynard JE, Lorenz D, Bradley DW. Review of infectivity studies in nonhuman primates with virus-like particles associated with MS-1 hepatitis. The American Journal of the Medical Sciences. 1975;**270**:81-85

[30] Andre FE, D'Hondt E, Delem A. Clinical assessment of the safety and efficacy of an inactivated hepatitis A vaccine: Rationale and summary of findings. Vaccine. 1992;**10**(1):160-168

[31] Ordman CW, Jennings CG, Janeway CA. Chemical, clinical, and immunological studies on the products of human plasma fractionation. XII. Use of concentrated normal human serum gamma globulin (human immune serum globulin) in the prevention and attenuation of measles. Journal of Clinical Investigation. 1944;**23**:541-549

[32] Stokes J, Neefe JR. The prevention and attenuation of infectious hepatitis with gamma globulin (preliminary note). JAMA. 1945;**127**:144-145

[33] Werzberger A, Mensch B, Kuter B, Brown L, Lewis J, Sitrin R, et al. A controlled trial of a formalin-inactivated hepatitis a vaccine in healthy children. The New England Journal of Medicine. 1992;**327**:453-457

[34] Innis BL, Snitbhan R, Kunasol P, Laorakpongse T, Poopatanakool W, Kozik CA, et al. Protection against hepatitis A by an inactivated vaccine. JAMA. 1994;**271**:1328-1334

[35] Sjogren MH, Hoke CH, Binn LN, Eckels KH, Dubois DR, Lyde L, et al. Immunogenicity of an inactivated hepatitis A vaccine. Annals of Internal Medicine. 1991;**114**:470-471

[36] Midthun K, Ellerbeck E, Gershman K, Calandra G, Krah D,

Mc-Caughtry M, et al. Safety and immunogenicity of a live attenuated hepatitis A virus vaccine in seronegative volunteers. The Journal of Infectious Diseases. 1991;**163**:735-739

[37] Shouval D. The immunological basis for immunization series. In: Immunization Vaccines and Biologicals. Switzerland: World Health Organization Department of Immunization; 2010. p. 39

[38] Cui F, Liang X, Wang F, Zheng H, Hutin YJ, Yang W. Development, production, and postmarketing surveillance of hepatitis A vaccines in China. Journal of Epidemiology. 2014;**24**:169-177

[39] Sabanin IV, Rikhter VV, Kuzin SN. Assessment of effectiveness and immunogenicity of hepatitis A vaccination in servicemen of internal forces of Ministry of Internal Affairs of Russia. Zhurnal Mikrobiologii, Epidemiologii, i Immunobiologii. 2010;**1**:35-39

[40] Gardner P, Eickhoff T, Poland GA, Gross P, Griffin M, LaForce FM, et al. Adult immunizations. Annals of Internal Medicine. 1996;**124**:35-40

[41] Iorio N, John S. Hepatitis A NCBI Bookshelf. A Service of the National Library of Medicine, National Institutes of Health. StatPearls [Internet]. Treasure Island (FL): StatPearls Publishing; 2019

[42] Gingrich GA, Hadler SC, Elder HA. Serologic investigation of an outbreak of hepatitis A in a rural day-care cente. American Journal of Public Health. 1983;**73**:1190-1193

[43] Verma R, Khanna P. Hepatitis A vaccine should receive priority in National Immunization Schedule in India. Human Vaccines & Immunotherapeutics. 2012;**8**(8):1132-1134

[44] Waszczuk K, Waszczuk E, Szenborn L. Can we better protect patients with inflammatory bowel disease against infections patient attitude and personal immunization knowledge. Acta Gastroenterologica Belgica. 2018;**81**(2):257-261

[45] O'Leary ST, Kimberlin DW. Update from the advisory committee on immunization practices. Journal of the Pediatric Infectious Diseases Society. 2018;**7**(3):181-187

[46] Singh V, Crosby RA, Gratzer B, Gorbach PM, Markowitz LE, Meites E. Disclosure of sexual behavior is significantly associated with receiving a panel of health care services recommended for men who have sex with men. Sexually Transmitted Diseases. 2018;**45**(12):803-807

[47] Groseclose SL, Brathwaite WS, Hall PA, Adams DA, Connor FJ, Sharp P, et al. Centers for Disease Control and Prevention. Summary of notifiable diseases, United States, 2000. MMWR Morbidity and Mortality Weekly Report. 2002;**49**:1-102

[48] Centers for Disease Control and Prevention. Hepatitis Surveil- lance Report No. 58. Atlanta; 2003

[49] Wasley A, Feinstone SM, Bell BP. Hepatitis A. In: Mandell GL, Bennett JE, Dolin R, editors. Mandell, Douglas, and Bennett's Principles and Practice of Infectious Diseases. 7th ed. Philadelphia: Churchill Livingstone; 2011. pp. 2367-2387

[50] Bell BP, Kruszon-Moran D, Shapiro CN. Hepatitis a virus infection in the United States: Serologic results from the third National Health and nutrition examination survey. Vaccine. 2005;**23**:5793-5806

[51] Mathur P, Arora N. Epidemiological transition of hepatitis A in India: Issues for vaccination in developing countries. Indian Journal of Medical Research. 2008;**128**(6):699-704

[52] Mantovani SAS, Delfino BM, Martins AC, Oliart-Guzmán H, Pereira TM, Branco FLCC, et al. Socioeconomic inequities and hepatitis A virus infection in Western Brazilian Amazonian children: Spatial distribution and associated factors. BMC Infectious Diseases. 2015;**15**(1):428

[53] Cooksley WG. What did we learn from the Shanghai hepatitis A epidemic? Journal of Viral Hepatitis. 2000;**7**(1):1-3

[54] World Health Organization. Hepatitis A Fact sheet No. 328. Available from: http://www.searo.who.int/thailand/factsheets/fs0030/en/ [Accessed: 31 July 2019]

[55] Mohd Hanafiah K, Jacobsen KH, Wiersma ST. Challenges to mapping the health risk of hepatitis A virus infection. International Journal of Health Geographics. 2011;**10**:57

[56] Barzaga BN. Hepatitis a, shifting epidemiology in South-East Asia and in China. Vaccine. 2000;**18**(1):61-64

[57] Poovorawan Y, Theamboonlers A, Sinalaparatsamee S, Chaiear K, Siraprapasiri T, Khwanjaipanich S, et al. Increasing susceptibility to HAV among members of the young generation in Thailand. Asian Pacific Journal of Allergy and Immunology. 2000;**18**:249-253

[58] Tanaka J. Hepatitis a shifting epidemiology in Latin America. Vaccine. 2000;**18**(1):57-60

[59] Sohn YM, Rho HO, Park MS. The changing epidemiology of hepatitis A in children and the consideration of active immunisation in Korea. Yonsei Medical Journal. 2000;**41**:34-39

[60] Dal-Re R, Garcia-Corberia P, Garcia-de-Lomas J. A large percentage of the Spanish population under 30 years of age is not protected against hepatitis A. Journal of Medical Virology. 2000;**60**:363-366

[61] Gdalvich M, Grotto I, Mandel Y, Mimouni D, Sherman J, Ashkenezi I. Hepatitis A antibody prevalence among young adults in Israel, the decline continues. Epidemiology and Infection. 1998;**1221**:477-479

[62] European Centre for Disease Prevention and Control. Annual Epidemiological Report Hepatitis A. Available from: https://ecdc.europa.eu/en/publications-data/hepatitis-annual-epidemiological-report-2016 [Accessed: 31 July 2019]

[63] Gozlan Y, Bar-Or I, Rakovsky A. Ongoing hepatitis A among men who have sex with men (MSM) linked to outbreaks in Europe in Tel Aviv area, Israel, December 2016–June 2017. Euro Surveillance. 2017;**22**:30575

[64] Klevens RM, Kruszon-Moran D, Wasley A. Seroprevalence of hepatitis A virus antibodies in the U.S.: Results from the National Health and nutrition examination survey. Public Health Reports. 2011;**126**:522-532

[65] Ly KN, Klevens RM. Trends in disease and complications of hepatitis A virus infection in the United States, 1999-2011: A new concern for adults. The Journal of Infectious Diseases. 2015;**212**:176-182

[66] Ariyarathna N, Abeysena C. Sero-prevalence of viral hepatitis A in a district of Sri Lanka: A community based cross-sectional study. BMC Infectious Diseases. 2019;**19**:443

[67] Tan EM, Marcelin JR, Virk A. Pretravel counseling for immunocompromised travelers: A 12year singlecenter retrospective review. Infection, Disease & Health. 2019;**24**(1):13-22

[68] CDC. Viral hepatitis surveillance Atlanta, GA: US Department of

Health and Human Service. Available from: https://www.cdc.gov/hepatitis/statistics/2016surveillance/pdfs/2016HepSurveillanceRpt.pdf [Accessed: 01 August 2019]

[69] CDC. Hepatitis surveillance: Report no. 55. Atlanta, GA: US Department of Health and Human. Available from: Service https://babel.hathitrust.org/cgi/pt?id=mdp.39015026224173;view=1up;seq=24 [Accessed: 01 August]

[70] Groseclose SL, Brathwaite WS, Hall PA, Adams DA, Connor FJ, Sharp P, et al. Centers for Disease Control Prevention. Summary of notifiable diseases, United States. MMWR Morbidity and Mortality Weekly Report. 2002;**49**:1-102

[71] Wasley A, Grytdal S, Gallagher K. Surveillance for acute viral hepatitis—United States, 2006. MMWR Surveillance Summaries. 2008;**57**:1-24

[72] Centers for Disease Control Prevention. Viral hepatitis surveillance, United States 2016. Atlanta, GA: US Department of Health and Human Services, CDC. Available from: https://www.cdc.gov/hepatitis/statistics/2016surveillance/pdfs/2016HepSurveillanceRpt.pdf [Accessed: 01 August 2019]

[73] Lagarde E, Joussemet M, Lataillade J, Fabre G. Risk factors for hepatitis A infection in France: Drinking tap water may be of importance. European Journal of Epidemiology. 1995;**11**(2):145-148

[74] Yun H, Lee HJ, Yoon Y, Kim K, Kim S, Shin MH, et al. Seroprevalence of hepatitis-antibodies in relation to social factors, a preliminary study. Osong Public Health and Research Perspectives. 2012;**3**(1):31-35

[75] Kiyohara T, Sato T, Totsuka A, Miyamura T, Ito T, Yoneyama T. Shifting Seroepidemiology of hepatitis A in Japan, 1973-2003. Microbiology and Immunology. 2007;**51**(2):185-191

[76] Tseng YT, Sun HY, Chang SY, Wu CH, Liu WC, Wu PY, et al. Seroprevalence of hepatitis virus infection in men who have sex with men aged 18-40 years in Taiwan. Journal of the Formosan Medical Association. 2012;**111**(8):431-438

[77] Lee YL, Lin KY, Cheng CY, Li CW, Yang CJ, Tsai MS, et al. Taiwan HIV study group. Evolution of hepatitis A virus seroprevalence among HIV-positive adults in Taiwan. PLoS One. 2017;**12**(10):e0186338. DOI: 10.1371/journal.pone.0186338

[78] Battegay M, Gust ID, Feinstone SM. Hepatitis A virus. In: Mandel JL, Bennett JE, editors. Principles and Practices of Infectious Diseases. New York: Churchill Livingstone; 1995. pp. 1636-1656

[79] Prince AM, Brotman B, Richardson L, White T, Pollock N, Riddle J. Incidence of hepatitis A virus (HAV) infection in rural Liberia. Journal of Medical Virology. 1985;**15**:421-428

[80] Brown P, Greguer G, Smallwood L, Ney R, Moerdowo RM, Gerety RJ. Serological markers of hepatitis A and B in the population of Bali, Indonesia. American Journal of Tropical Medicine and Hygiene. 1985;**34**:616-619

[81] Tandon BN, Gandhi BM, Joshi YK. Etiological spectrum of viral hepatitis and prevalence of markers of hepatitis A and B virus in northern India. Bulletin of the World Health Organization. 1984;**62**:67-73

[82] Das K, Jain A, Gupta S, Kapoor S, Gupta RK, Chakravorty A, et al. The changing epidemiological pattern of hepatitis A virus in an urban population in India: Emergence of a trend similar to

European countries. European Journal of Epidemiology. 2000;**16**:507-510

[83] Dhawan PS, Shah SS, Alvares JF, Kher A, Shankaran KPW, et al. Seroprevalence of hepatitis A virus in Mumbai and immunogenicity and safety of hepatitis A vaccine. Indian Journal of Gastroenterology. 1998;**17**:16-18

[84] Das K, Kar P, Chakarborty A, Gupta S, Das BC. Is a vaccination programme against hepatitis A needed in India? Indian Journal of Gastroenterology. 1998;**17**:158

[85] Arankalle V, Mitra M, Bhave S. Changing epidemiology of hepatitis A virus in Indian children. Dovepress. 2014;**4**:7-13

[86] Aggarwal R, Naik S, Yachha SK, Naik SR. Seroprevalence of antibodies to the hepatitis A virus among children in northern India. Indian Paediatrics. 1999;**36**:1248-1250

[87] Freidl GS, Sonder GJ, Bovée LP, Friesema IH, van Rijckevorsel GG, Ruijs WL, et al. Hepatitis A outbreak among men who have sex with men (MSM) predominantly linked with the EuroPride, the Netherlands, July 2016 to February 2017. Euro Surveillance. 2017;**22**(8):30468

[88] Acharya SK, Batra Y, Bhatkal B. Seroepidemiology of hepatitis A virus infection among school children in Delhi and north Indian patients with chronic liver disease: Implications for HAV vaccination. Journal of Gastroenterology and Hepatology. 2003;**18**(7):822-827

[89] Fix AD, Martin OS, Gallicchio L, Vial PA, Lagos R. Age-specific prevalence of antibodies to hepatitis A in Santiago, Chile: Risk factors and shift in age of infection among children and young adults. The American Journal of Tropical Medicine and Hygiene. 2002;**66**(5):628-632

[90] Acharya SK, Madan K, Dattagupta S, Panda SK. Viral hepatitis in India. National Medical Journal of India. 2006;**19**(4):203-217

[91] Hayajneh WA, Balbeesi A, Faouri S. Hepatitis A virus age-specific sero- prevalence and risk factors among Jordanian children. Journal of Medical Virology. 2015;**87**(4):569-574

[92] Centers for Disease Control and Prevention. Morbidity and Mortality Weekly Report (MMWR). Provisional cases of selected notifiable diseases, and selected low frequency diseases, United States and U.S. territories, weeks ending November 11, 2017, and November 12, 2016. Available from: www.cdc.gov/mmwr/volumes/66/wr/mm6645md.htm [Accessed: 01 August 2019]

[93] Centers for Disease Control and Prevention. Viral hepatitis: 2016–Multistate outbreak of hepatitis A linked to frozen strawberries (final update). Available from: www.cdc.gov/hepatitis/outbreaks/2016/hav-strawberries.htm [Accessed: 28 July 2019]

[94] State of Hawaii, Department of Health: Disease Outbreak Control Division. Hepatitis A outbreak 2016. Available from: http://health.hawaii.gov/docd/hepatitis-a-outbreak-2016 [Accessed: 28 July 2019]

[95] California Department of Public Health. Hepatitis A outbreak in California. 2018. Available from: www.cdph.ca.gov/Programs/CID/DCDC/Pages/Immunization/Hepatitis-A-Outbreak.aspx [Accessed: 28 July 2019]

[96] Donnan EJ, Fielding JE, Gregory JE, Lalor K, Rowe S, Goldsmith P, et al. A multistate outbreak of hepatitis A associated with semidried tomatoes in

Australia. Clinical Infectious Diseases. 2012;**54**:775-781

[97] Integrated Disease Surveillance Project. Recent Weekly Outbreak. Available from: http://www.idsp.nic.in/index4.php?lang=1&level=0&linkid=406&lid=3689 [Last Accessed: 01 August 2019]

[98] Rakesh PS, Mainu TT, Raj A, Babu D, Rajiv M, Sreelakshmi K, et al. Investigating a community wide outbreak of hepatitis A in Kerala, India. Journal of Family Medicine and Primary Care. 2018;7:1537-1541

[99] Jain P, Prakash S, Gupta S. Prevalence of hepatitis A virus, hepatitis B virus, hepatitis C virus, hepatitis D virus and hepatitis E virus as causes of acute viral hepatitis in North India: A hospital based study. Indian Journal of Medical Microbiology. 2013;**31**(3):261-265

[100] Arankalle VA, Sarada Devi KL, Lole KS, Shenoy KT, Verma V, Haneephabi M. Molecular characterization of hepatitis A virus from a large outbreak from Kerala, India. Indian Journal of Medical Research. 2006;**123**(6):760-769

[101] Rakesh PS, Sherin D, Sankar H, Shaji M, Subhagan S, Salila S. Investigating a community-wide outbreak of hepatitis A in India. Journal of Global Infectious Diseases. 2014;**6**(2):59-64

[102] Gassowski M, Michaelis K, Wenzel JJ, Faber M, Figoni J, Mouna L, et al. Two concurrent outbreaks of hepatitis A highlight the risk of infection for non-immune travellers to Morocco, January to June 2018. Euro Surveillance. 2018;**5**(27):1-5

[103] Latash J, Dorsinville M, Del Rosso P, Antwi M, Reddy V, Waechter H, et al. Notes from the eld: increase in reported hepatitis a infections among men who have sex with men - New York City, January-August 2017. MMWR Morbidity and Mortality Weekly Report. 2017;**66**(37):999-1000. DOI: 10.15585/mmwr.mm6637a7

[104] Urbanus AT, van Houdt R, van de Laar TJ, Coutinho RA. Viral hepatitis among men who have sex with men, epidemiology and public health consequences. Euro Surveillance. 2009;**14**(47):19-21

[105] Stene-Johansen K, Tjon G, Schreier E, Bremer V, Bruisten S, Ngui SL, et al. Molecular epidemiological studies show that hepatitis A virus is endemic among active homosexual men in Europe. Journal of Medical Virology. 2007;**79**(4):356-365

[106] Edelstein M, Turbitt D, Balogun K, Figueroa J, Nixon G. Hepatitis A outbreak in an orthodox Jewish community in London, July 2010. Eurosurveillance. 2010;**15**(37):19662

[107] Lim HS, Choi K, Lee S. Epidemiological investigation of an outbreak of hepatitis A at a residential facility for the disabled. Journal of Preventive Medicine and Public Health. 2013;**46**(2):62-73

[108] European Centre for Disease Prevention and Control (ECDC). Rapid risk assessment: Hepatitis A outbreak in the EU/EEA mostly affecting men who have sex with men. Available from: https://ecdc.europa.eu/en/publications-data/rapid-risk-assessment-hepatitis-outbreak-eueea-mostly-affecting-men-who-have-sex [Accessed: 28 July 2019]

Chapter 2

Hepatitis A: At-Risk Populations

Rosa Coelho and Guilherme Macedo

Abstract

Hepatitis A virus (HAV) is transmitted mostly through exposure to contaminated food or water, or through exposure to infected persons. This infection can occur sporadically or in an epidemic form, confers lifelong immunity and it is preventable by a safe and effective vaccine. Therefore, prevention strategies are crucial and could eradicate the infection if they were successfully employed. In this chapter, authors summarize mode of transmission and preventive measures for HAV among the following population groups: travellers, health care workers, men who have sex with men, individuals who use illicit drugs, sewage workers, food handlers, military personnel, prisoners, blood transfusions recipients, haemophiliacs and patients with HIV and chronic liver disease. Moreover, authors describe which of these groups are eligible for HAV vaccination according to available data.

Keywords: hepatitis A, MSM, men who have sex with men, outbreak, sexually transmitted infections, viral infections, viral infections

1. Introduction

Hepatitis A virus (HAV) is a common cause of acute viral hepatitis and caused approximately 11 000 deaths in 2015 worldwide (accounting for 0.8% of the mortality from viral hepatitis) [1].

HAV infection can occur sporadically or in an epidemic form, confers lifelong immunity [2] and is preventable by a safe and effective vaccine. As a matter of fact, humans are the only known reservoir for HAV, so the successful employment of widespread prevention strategies could eradicate the infection.

In the literature, some risk groups for HAV infection were identified, such as travellers, healthcare workers (HCWs), men who have sex with men (MSM), individuals who use illicit drugs, sewage workers, food handlers, military personnel, prisoners, blood transfusions recipients and haemophiliacs [3].

2. Mode of transmission

HAV is usually transmitted by the faecal-oral route: primarily through close personal contact or by oral intake after faecal contamination of skin or mucous membranes. Less commonly, the transmission occurs due to consumption of contaminated food or water [4].

Regarding person to person contact, the transmission can occur within households, residential institutions and daycare centres, among military personnel and during sexual intercourse. HAV infection due to consumption of contaminated food or water includes ingesting raw or undercooked foods, namely, shellfish and vegetables, or consumption of meals contaminated by infected food handlers.

Other modes of HAV transmission are due to blood transfusion and use of illicit drugs. Maternal-foetal transmission has not been described.

According to endemicity of hepatitis A (HA) disease, it can occur in three distinct ways [5]. In developing countries, with poor sanitary infrastructure, there are high infection rates occurring in childhood, and HA is endemic. Therefore, in these areas outbreaks are not frequent, and children develop immunity without ever being symptomatic [5]. In contrast, in developed countries with adequate sanitation and infrastructure, infection rates are low, and outbreaks are infrequent as long as the disease is not introduced into the population from an external source [5, 6]. Countries with intermediate levels of HA present increased numbers of susceptible adults and, occasionally, large outbreaks [5, 7]. In terms of HA endemicity, it is important to point out that exportation of food that cannot be sterilised, from countries of high endemicity to areas with low rates of infection, is a potentially important source of infection [5–7].

3. At-risk populations

3.1 Travellers to endemic countries

Travel is still one of the most important risk factors for HAV infection despite the improvement of socio-economic level considering the last decades [8]. The risk is varied and depends on the endemicity of visited countries and on the adherence of hygienic practices [3, 8].

Although the risk of infection may have slightly decreased in recent years, the incidence rate for non-protected travellers is estimated to be 3 cases per 1000 travellers per month of stay in developing countries [3].

A population-based study performed showed that the highest risk was associated with travel to East Africa followed by the Middle East, India and neighbouring countries [9]. The risk increases among young children visiting friends and relatives that accounted for a large proportion of cases and should be prioritised for vaccination [8, 10].

Few prevalence studies with contrasting and inconclusive data have been published regarding anti-HAV positivity and history of travel [3].

Considering prophylaxis for travellers in several countries, many recommendations and guidelines have been issued emphasising the importance of a correct information and prophylaxis for this at-risk group. Bearing in mind that vaccinated travellers still represent a small amount, it is crucial to promote this prophylaxis measure among physicians and this at-risk population [3].

3.2 Men who have sex with men

Since the 1980s, when an important decrease in HA incidence due to socio-economic improvements was evident, a peak in the incidence of HAV was noticed in males from 20 to 39 years old. These cases were attributed to sexually transmitted HAV and justified some outbreaks among MSM that have been described in Denmark, Sweden, the United Kingdom and the United States [3, 11, 12]. The predominant circulating HAV strains among MSM belonged to genotype IA [13].

Among MSM population, some risk factors for HAV infection were identified, such as oro-anal sexual practices and digital-rectal intercourse, history of sexual contacts with anonymous sex partners, group sex and sexual promiscuity [3].

As a matter of fact, in this at-risk group, the widespread availability and use of mobile-accessible, especially geosocial networking apps for MSM facilitate anonymous sexual activities being potential drivers of recent outbreaks of HAV [13–16]. On the other hand, dating apps and websites can be an important and effective tool to promote HAV infection prevention campaigns in outbreaks, with the advantage of a range of hard-to-reach MSM seeking anonymous sex [17].

Although MSM with sexual behaviour risks are responsible for HAV infection outbreaks, several prevalence studies do not demonstrate significant differences in anti-HAV positivity between MSM and control groups (general population/persons who use illicit drugs) [3].

Since the mid-1990s, HAV vaccine has been licenced and recommended for MSM. However, the emergence of HAV infection has continued to constitute a health threat to MSM in several developed countries [13].

3.3 Persons who use illicit drugs

Since the 1970s, as the numbers of injecting drug users (IDUs) increased, several outbreaks of acute HAV infection among IDUs' communities have been reported in several developed countries of low endemicity for HAV infection [13].

HAV acute infection in this at-risk group is strongly associated with the changing prevalence of this viral infection in the general population, usually in whom natural immunity was reduced in countries with low incidence.

Most of the outbreaks were described in Europe and the United States in the 1980s and 1990s but were seldom described after the early 2000s [13]. Some prevalence studies described an increased antibody prevalence among IDUs [3].

Transmission can occur via faecal-oral contact through poor personal hygiene and living conditions or percutaneously through contamination of illicit drugs or injecting equipment by faecal materials or blood [13, 18].

In the literature the most important risk factors identified for HAV infection in this group are scarce personal hygiene, socio-economic factors, sexual promiscuity, syringe exchange and contamination of instruments used to prepare drug consumption [3].

Prevention of HAV is important, and vaccination programmes should be implemented as occurred already in some European countries, such as the United Kingdom, Norway and Italy [13].

3.4 Food handlers

In the HAV transmission chain, food handlers can be involved in two different ways: they can become infected via contaminated food (principally shellfish and raw seafood), and, once infected, they may be the source of outbreaks [3].

Despite numerous HAV epidemics having been described [3], since the introduction of the HAV vaccine, the incidence of HAV infection has decreased, including those among food handlers [19].

However, due to their occupation, food handlers are not considered an at-risk group for HAV infection, as it can be easily avoidable if the most common hygienic precautions are taken. Some studies described a very slight increase in prevalence in food handlers under the age of 30 years versus the general population of the same age. Also higher anti-HAV antibody seroprevalence was detected in the personnel employed in the kitchen than in medical personnel, but socio-economic factors are not taken into account [3]. Nonetheless, this group may belong to demographic groups, such as young people and people with lower socio-economic status, who have a higher incidence of HAV than the general population [20].

Mandatory food handler vaccination is unlikely to be cost-effective. However, based on local needs, health departments of each country should make decisions about requiring vaccination for this group [21].

3.5 Healthcare workers

Data regarding the mode of HAV transmission show that personal contact with an infected person is the most common risk factor for developing the infection. Thus, healthcare workers are at potential risk of exposure to contagious patients infected with HA, particularly in paediatric wards [22–24].

The analysis of several studies regarding outbreaks in hospital settings indicates the main risk factors are eating and drinking in hospital divisions and inadequate hand cleaning [3].

The seroprevalence studies did not show consistent findings, and there were wide variations in the proportion of seropositive HCWs, taking into account different countries and professional groups [24].

As a matter of fact, studies comparing anti-HAV antibody seroprevalence between paediatric divisions' nurses and nurses of other hospital departments did not show any difference [3].

It is interesting to point out that one study comparing the hospital laundry workers with nurses suggested that the former group was more exposed to HA occupational risk, probably due to contact with handling dirty linen prior to washing them [25].

However, considering that universal precautions should be implemented in healthcare centres, some authors might argue that HCWs do not constitute an at-risk group for HAV [3, 24].

Nonetheless, considering that HA vaccines provide a safe, immunogenic and efficacious prevention tool, some authors recommend vaccination considering that HCWs are exposed to a higher risk infection than the general population [24].

It is crucial to implement general precautionary measures at the workplace that could reduce the transmission of HAV. Moreover, it is crucial that hospitals have an effective infection control of HA outbreaks which means early recognition, including awareness of atypical presentations of HAV infection, and strict adherence to universal infection control measures [24].

3.6 Sewage workers

Wastewater plant workers may be exposed to various infectious agents. However, at the moment it is unclear whether sewage workers have an increased risk of contracting HA or not, especially if the disease is preventable by using a vaccine [26].

Actually, sewage workers can be exposed to aerosols and direct contact with potentially contaminated materials such as raw wastewater, which means that a plausible biological risk to acquire HA in this group of employees exists [3, 26]. However, studies regarding anti-HAV antibody seroprevalence and risk of acquiring the disease are conflicting [26]. A recent systematic review [27] concluded that the incidence of clinical HA does not show an increased risk in sewage workers. Nonetheless, it found a moderately increased risk of subclinical HA infection when seroprevalence studies are considered. Results of seroprevalence studies may be flawed by several methodological factors.

Considering these discrepant results, there is no consensus on the need to vaccinate sewage workers. On the one hand, some authors recommend a systematic vaccination because of the increased risk. On the other hand, some authors do not consider vaccination necessary, and some authors consider that vaccination programmes can be discussed for those workers heavily exposed to sewage [27].

Some specialists in occupational health just recommend immunisation in order to "maintain labour peace", to prevent litigation costs, or only after evaluating the specific epidemiological situation [27].

However, these conclusions may not be generalisable to populations with different natural immunity as they are based mostly on investigations from Europe and North America [27].

3.7 Military personnel

Control of HA has been an important concern for US military forces in war and peace mostly in the past. However, nowadays due to the improvement of the sanitation level with better hygienic sanitary conditions, the risk of HA in this group is mainly attributed to activities in high endemic areas. As a matter of fact, this group usually works in difficult areas characterised by poor hygienic conditions and scarce control on food sources and drinking water supplies. Moreover, in remote areas, soldiers can be exposed to parenterally transmitted infections in case of injuries, hospitalisations and transfusions [3, 28]. In fact, most studies reporting HA epidemics among military personnel were published before 1990 showing numerous HA outbreaks that devastated whole army forces during the world wars, conditioning the military strategies [3].

Almost all the studies published later analysed the vaccine effectiveness and suggest different vaccination programmes considering soldiers as an at-risk group for HA [3].

However, in several papers military personnel is considered just as a sample of the general population, and as it has been recently occurring in other groups, a decrease in seroprevalence is evident. Moreover, only a few studies analyse the correlation between HA infection with epidemiologic factors such as overcrowding and consumption of contaminated food and water in military activities [3].

A recent and large multicentric cross-sectional study (11 training centres) conducted within the Indian Armed Forces during 1 year (2010–2011) showed a high seroprevalence of HAV (93%) among healthy young adults [29]. In contrast, HA was found to be a cause of acute viral hepatitis in 30% of 102 cases seen in an Armed Forces hospital from southern India [30]. So, even in the same countries, data are not consistent, and therefore, it can be difficult to justify the economic cost of universal HAV vaccination.

3.8 Prisoners

Prison is considered to be an environment where many risk factors for HA can be easily identified, such as overcrowding, frequent prison relocation, sexual promiscuity, drug abuse and poor sanitation.

As a matter of fact, prison facilities in which inmates live in close proximity and engage in high-risk behaviours for HAV transmissions may diminish the effectiveness of strategies of infection control based on universal adoption of hygienic practices [31].

Data regarding HAV prevalence among prisoners are few, conflicting and not conclusive [3]. Epidemiological investigations concluded that HA among prisoners have been introduced mainly by newly arrived prison entrants who were incarcerated during their incubation period who subsequently developed acute HA [31].

A recent cross-sectional survey undertaken after a multicentre outbreak of HAV infection in the Queensland prison system, following a community-based HAV epidemic among users of illicit drugs, identifies the determinants for recent and past HAV infection [31]. The authors concluded that the common factor among recently acquired and past infection of HA was due to the use of illicit drugs. In contrast, there was no evidence that IDUs were associated to higher rates of HAV-IgG seropositivity (past infection) [31].

In prison settings, routine vaccination of all susceptible inmates with inactivated HA vaccine may be considered as an important strategy in order to prevent transmission of HAV infection especially during periods of higher incidence among the incoming prisoner population [31].

3.9 Blood transfusion recipients

HAV infection is not a significant complication of blood transfusion due to the short-lasting viremic period [3]. As a matter of fact, considering the sporadic nature of the HAV acute infection among blood donors and the lack of HAV chronic carriers, antibody screening tests for HAV for serological screening of blood donors are not recommended in any country [32]. However, even if it is rare, HAV parenteral transmission is possible, and many countries recommend vaccination for polytransfused patients [33, 34].

In the past, some epidemic cases of HA were reportedly caused by children who received infected blood or plasma. However, none of the prospective studies, conducted in the 1970s and 1980s to establish incidence and agents of posttransfusion hepatitis, identified cases of HAV infection [3]. In fact, no data showing higher prevalence of HAV in subjects receiving blood transfusion are available, which means that there is no evidence to consider polytransfused patients as a risk group.

Nonetheless, recently two cases of HAV transmission to blood recipients from a healthy donor that later presented to the blood bank with jaundice were published [32]. Actually, one of the cases was fatal and the patient died from fulminant HA. It is important to highlight that the patient was immunocompromised due to bone marrow transplantation and had also hepatitis C [32]. This case report points out the importance of timely identification of post-donation symptoms and notification to blood banks and also that specific groups of immunocompromised patients may benefit from a HAV vaccination programme [32].

3.10 Haemophiliacs

Some outbreaks of HAV infection among haemophilia patients have been reported due to transfusions of factors VIII/IX concentrates treated with the solvent/detergent method used to inactivate blood-borne viruses [3]. In fact, in these studies a causal relationship was found between the injection of blood clotting factors and an outbreak of HA among haemophilia patients.

Clotting factor concentrates manufactured from large pool may be contaminated by HAV, which can be present even in a single highly viremic blood donor.

The solvent/detergent method used to inactivate HAV virus seemed to be not effective to ensure the safety of clotting factor concentrates [35]. Therefore, Guilaume TA et al. proposed a new method using a terminal 100°C dry-heat sterilisation in order to destroy also non-lipid-enveloped viruses [36].

However, case–control papers and studies regarding seroprevalence of HAV in this group did not show an increased risk of contracting HA among haemophiliacs [3], and therefore at present haemophiliacs are not included as an at-risk group to acquire HAV.

3.11 Other populations

HA results in acute liver failure in less than 1%, age superior to 50 years old and those with underlying liver disease being important risk factors, especially with chronic hepatitis B and C virus infections [37, 38]. As a matter of fact, HAV superinfection in patients with underlying chronic liver disease is not also associated with a high risk of liver failure but also of death [37, 38].

Besides, patients with pre-existing liver disease (i.e. non-alcoholic fatty liver disease or alcoholic steatohepatitis) present a higher risk of developing an acute-on-chronic liver failure in cases of HAV infection [38, 39].

Therefore, it has been recommended to vaccinate against HAV in patients with chronic liver disease [40]. Nonetheless, studies show HAV testing and vaccination rates were low in clinical practice. Public health programmes are needed in order to increase awareness about HAV vaccination in patients with pre-existing liver damage [41–43].

HAV infections among older individuals continue to pose public health and clinical challenges because HA illness severity increases with age, presence of liver disease and other comorbid medical conditions [42]. In fact, the increased number of HAV infection in hospitalised patients with hypertension, ischemic heart disease, disorders of lipid metabolism and chronic kidney disease may also reflect increasing age. Older age (over 65 years old) and any liver disease are independent risk factors to being hospitalised more than 5 days, suggesting that these factors increase the severity of HA illness [42]. Therefore, more studies are needed to guide recommendations for HA vaccination in adults with other chronic diseases other than chronic liver disease.

Considering HIV-positive individuals, only very few studies with a limit number of patients address the risk of HA in these populations [3]. Even though the direct evidence on the correlation between contracting HIV and HAV was scarce, observational data suggested that HIV-positive individuals, especially MSM and IDUs, are at increased risk of acquiring HAV [3]. Moreover, Ida et al. published a study of 15 HIV-positive individuals that showed that the duration of HAV viremia in HIV-seropositive individuals with acute HA was prolonged compared to that in HIV-negative individuals, which may increase the probability of HAV transmission to others [44].

Considering HIV-seropositive patients, two independent risk factors associated with seropositivity for HAV were recognised: older age and injecting drug use. However, HAV seroprevalence was lower in HIV-positive MSM despite the at-risk sexual behaviours [13].

Regarding prophylaxis in HIV-positive patients, HAV vaccination is not universally recommended but specifically for those with increased risks of exposure (such as from injecting drug use, oral-anal sex, travel to or residence in endemic areas, frequent clotting factor or blood transfusions) or with increased risks of fulminant disease (such as those with chronic hepatitis) [45, 46].

Author details

Rosa Coelho and Guilherme Macedo*
Gastroenterology Department, Centro Hospitalar São João, Porto, Portugal

*Address all correspondence to: guilhermemacedo59@gmail.com

References

[1] Hepatitis A fact sheet. In: World Health Organization: Media centre. [website] http://www.who.int/mediacentre/factsheets/fs328/en/

[2] Cuthbert JA. Hepatitis A: Old and new. Clinical Microbiology Reviews. 2001;**14**(1):38-58

[3] Franco E, Giambi C, Ialacci R, Coppola RC, Zanetti AR. Risk groups for hepatitis A virus infection. Vaccine. 2003;**21**(19-20):2224-2233

[4] Daniels D, Grytdal S, Wasley A, Centers for Disease Control and Prevention (CDC). Surveillance for acute viral hepatitis—United States, 2007. MMWR Surveillance Summaries. 2009;**58**(3):1

[5] Shapiro CN, Margolis HS. Worldwide epidemiology of hepatitis A virus infection. Journal of Hepatology. 1993;**18**(Suppl 2):S11-S14

[6] Klevens RM, Denniston MM, Jiles-Chapman RB, Murphy TV. Decreasing immunity to hepatitis A virus infection among US adults: Findings from the National Health and nutrition examination survey (NHANES), 1999-2012. Vaccine. 2015;**33**(46):6192-6198

[7] Hofmeister MG, Foster MA, Teshale EH. Epidemiology and transmission of hepatitis A virus and hepatitis E virus infections in the United States. Cold Spring Harbor Perspectives in Medicine. 2019;**9**(4):pii: a033431

[8] Beauté J, Westrell T, Schmid D, et al. Travel-associated hepatitis A in Europe, 2009 to 2015. Euro Surveillance. 2018;**23**(22):1700583

[9] Askling HH, Rombo L, Andersson Y, Martin S, Ekdahl K. Hepatitis A risk in travelers. Journal of Travel Medicine. 2009;**16**(4):233-238

[10] Sane J, de Sousa R, van Pelt W, Petrignani M, Verhoef L, Koopmans M. Risk of hepatitis A decreased among Dutch travelers to endemic regions in 2003 to 2011. Journal of Travel Medicine. 2015;**22**(3):208-211

[11] Mazick A, Howitz M, Rex S, et al. Hepatitis A outbreak among MSM linked to casual sex and gay saunas in Copenhagen, Denmark. Euro Surveillance. 2005;**10**(5):5-6

[12] Sfetcu O, Irvine N, Ngui SL, Emerson C, McCaughey C, Donaghy P. Hepatitis A outbreak predominantly affecting men who have sex with men in Northern Ireland, October 2008 to July 2009. Euro Surveillance. 2011;**16**(9):16

[13] Lin KY, Chen GJ, Lee YL, et al. Hepatitis A virus infection and hepatitis A vaccination in human immunodeficiency virus-positive patients: A review. World Journal of Gastroenterology. 2017;**23**(20):3589-3606

[14] Thomas DR, Williams CJ, Andrady U, et al. Outbreak of syphilis in men who have sex with men living in rural North Wales (UK) associated with the use of social media. Sexually Transmitted Infections. 2016;**92**(5):359-364

[15] Beebeejaun K, Degala S, Balogun K, et al. Outbreak of hepatitis A associated with men who have sex with men (MSM), England, July 2016 to January 2017. Euro Surveillance. 2 Feb 2017;**22**(5). DOI: 10.2807/1560-7917.ES.2017.22.5.30454

[16] Gilbart VL, Simms I, Jenkins C, et al. Sex, drugs and smart phone applications: Findings from semistructured interviews with men who have sex with men diagnosed with Shigella flexneri 3a in England and Wales. Sexually Transmitted Infections. 2015;**91**(8):598-602

[17] Ruscher C, Werber D, Thoulass J, et al. Dating apps and websites as tools to reach anonymous sexual contacts during an outbreak of hepatitis A among men who have sex with men, Berlin, 2017. Euro Surveillance. 2019;**24**(21):1800460

[18] Spada E, Genovese D, Tosti ME, et al. An outbreak of hepatitis A virus infection with a high case-fatality rate among injecting drug users. Journal of Hepatology. 2005;**43**(6):958-964

[19] Sharapov UM, Kentenyants K, Groeger J, Roberts H, Holmberg SD, Collier MG. Hepatitis A infections among food handlers in the United States, 1993-2011. Public Health Reports. 2016;**131**(1):26-29

[20] Fiore AE. Hepatitis A transmitted by food. Clinical Infectious Diseases. 2004;**38**(5):705-715. Epub 2004 Feb 11

[21] Meltzer MI, Shapiro CN, Mast EE, Arcari C. The economics of vaccinating restaurant workers against hepatitis A. Vaccine. 2001;**19**:2138-2145

[22] Shapiro CN, Coleman PJ, McQuillan GM, et al. Epidemiology of hepatitis A: Seroepidemiology and risk groups in the USA. Vaccine. 1992;**10**(Suppl):S59-S62

[23] Smith S, Weber S, Wiblin T, et al. Cost-effectiveness of hepatitis A vaccination in healthcare workers. Infection Control and Hospital Epidemiology. 1997;**18**:688-691

[24] Chodick G, Ashkenazi S, Lerman Y. The risk of hepatitis A infection among healthcare workers: A review of reported outbreaks and sero-epidemiologic studies. The Journal of Hospital Infection. 2006;**62**(4):414-420. Epub 2006 Feb 20

[25] Borg MA, Portelli A. Hospital laundry workers-an at-risk group for hepatitis A? Occupational Medicine (London). 1999;**49**(7):448-450

[26] Divizia M, Cencioni B, Palombi L, Panà A. Sewage workers: Risk of acquiring enteric virus infections including hepatitis A. The New Microbiologica. 2008;**31**(3):337-334

[27] Glas C, Hotz P, Steffen R. Hepatitis A in workers exposed to sewage: A systematic review. Occupational and Environmental Medicine. 2001;**58**(12):762-768

[28] Puri P, Sharma PK, Nagpal AK. Viral hepatitis in India: Armed forces perspective. Medical Journal, Armed Forces India. 2016;**72**(3):201-203

[29] Kotwal A, Singh H, Verma AK. A study of hepatitis A and E virus seropositivity profile amongst young healthy adults in India. Medical Journal, Armed Forces India. 2014;**70**:225-229

[30] Nandi B, Hadimani P, Srunachalam R, Ganjoo RK. Spectrum of acute viral hepatitis in southern India. Medical Journal, Armed Forces India. 2009;**65**:7-9

[31] Whiteman D, McCall B, Falconer A. Prevalence and determinants of hepatitis A virus exposure among prison entrants in Queensland, Australia: Implications for public health control. Journal of Viral Hepatitis. 1998;**5**(4):277-283

[32] Gonçalves S, Leon L, Alves G, et al. A rare case of transfusion transmission of hepatitis A virus to two patients with Haematological disease. Transfusion Medicine and Hemotherapy. 2016;**43**(2):137-141

[33] Anonymous. Workshop Consensus Conference, Roma, 1995. The Italian Journal of Gastroenterology. 1996;**28**:181-184

[34] Lagarder B. Vaccination contre l'hepatite A. Archives de Pédiatrie. 1998;**5**:321-325

[35] Lawlor E, Graham S, Davidson F, et al. Hepatitis A transmission by factor IX concentrates. Vox Sanguinis. 1996;**71**:126-128

[36] Guilaume TA. Outbreaks of hepatitis A and emergence of new AIDS-associated agents: The need to add terminal 100°C dry-heat sterilization to factor VIII and factor IX concentrates. Vox Sanguinis. 1993;**65**:158

[37] Wasley A, Fiore A, Bell BP. Hepatitis A in the era of vaccination. Epidemiologic Reviews. 2006;**28**:101-111. Epub 2006 Jun 14

[38] Mank P, Verheyen J, Gerken G, Canbaya A. Liver failure due to acute viral hepatitis (A-E). Visceral Medicine. 2016;**32**(2):80-85

[39] Canbay A, Chen SY, Gieseler RK, et al. Overweight patients are more susceptible for acute liver failure. Hepato-Gastroenterology. 2005-Oct;**52**(65):1516-1520

[40] Strikas RA, Centers for Disease Control and Prevention (CDC), Advisory Committee on Immunization Practices (ACIP), ACIP Child/Adolescent Immunization Work Group. Advisory Committee on immunization practices recommended immunization schedules for persons aged 0 through 18 years—United States. MMWR. Morbidity and Mortality Weekly Report. 2015;**64**(4):93

[41] Shim M, Khaykis I, Park J, Bini EJ. Susceptibility to hepatitis A in patients with chronic liver disease due to hepatitis C virus infection: Missed opportunities for vaccination. Hepatology. 2005;**42**(3):688-695

[42] Collier MG, Tong X, Xu F. Hepatitis A hospitalizations in the United States, 2002-2011. Hepatology. 2015;**61**(2):481-485

[43] CDC. Adult vaccination coverage—United States, 2010. MMWR. Morbidity and Mortality Weekly Report. 2012;**61**:66-72

[44] Ida S, Tachikawa N, Nakajima A, Daikoku M, Yano M, Kikuchi Y, et al. Influence of human immunodeficiency virus type 1 infection on acute hepatitis A virus infection. Clinical Infectious Diseases. 2002;**34**:379-385

[45] Aberg JA, Gallant JE, Ghanem KG, Emmanuel P, Zingman BS, Horberg MA. Primary care guidelines for the management of persons infected with HIV: 2013 update by the HIV medicine Association of the Infectious Diseases Society of America. Clinical Infectious Diseases. 2014;**58**(1):e1-e34

[46] Panel on Opportunistic Infections in HIV-Infected Adults and Adolescents. Guidelines for the prevention and treatment of opportunistic infections in HIV-infected adults and adolescents: Recommendations from the Centres for Disease Control and Prevention, The National Institutes of Health, and the HIV Medicine Association of the Infectious Diseases Society of America. 2018

Chapter 3

Epidemiological Aspects of Hepatitis A: Endemicity Patterns and Molecular Epidemiology

Saba Gargouri, Lamia Fki-Berrajah, Imen Ayadi, Amel Chtourou, Adnene Hammami and Héla Karray-Hakim

Abstract

Improvements in hygiene and socio-economic conditions in many parts of the world have led to an epidemiological shift in hepatitis A with a transition from high to low endemicity. Consequently, in these areas, higher proportion of symptomatic disease among adolescents resulting in large-scale community outbreaks has been described. In Tunisia, an increase in the average age at the time of infection has been reported, hence resulting in regular outbreaks, especially household and primary school epidemics. Molecular investigation of such outbreaks, based on the determination of viral genotype and genetic relatedness between hepatitis A virus (HAV) strains, is a useful tool to identify the potential source of HAV contamination but also to assess the virus molecular dynamics over time, such as the introduction of a new genotype or a specific clustering of HAV strains according to the geographical origin. In Sfax city, (Center-East of Tunisia), only HAV strains of genotype IA are circulating. In rural areas, HAV infection is still highly endemic with probably a water-borne transmission pattern. Nevertheless, the considerable genetic heterogeneity observed in urban areas highlights the changing pattern of hepatitis A epidemiology in these settings. Further molecular studies are strongly needed to better understand HAV epidemiology in Tunisia.

Keywords: hepatitis A virus, epidemiology, Tunisia, incidence, RT-PCR, phylogenetic analysis, genetic relatedness, genotype, outbreak

1. Introduction

Hepatitis A is the most common cause of acute viral hepatitis in the world. This acute necro-inflammatory process of the liver is due to a picornavirus transmitted by the fecal-oral route, which is the hepatitis A virus (HAV). The severity and the clinical outcome of hepatitis A are closely related to the age of infection, with older ages being at risk for symptomatic disease and even acute liver failure. Improvements in socioeconomic and hygienic conditions, during the two last decades, have led to a change in the epidemiology of HAV infection worldwide [1]. This change is associated with a great potential for outbreaks and an increase in the mortality rate due to HAV. Consequently, hepatitis A can currently represent a serious public health problem, especially in regions undergoing this epidemiological change. Thus, it is crucial to recognize this evolution in the HAV epidemiology, in order to implement adequate preventive measures. Currently, seroprevalence surveys of hepatitis A, in addition to molecular investigation of HAV strains, are very useful tools to assess HAV epidemiology in a given area in the world [2].

2. Endemicity patterns of hepatitis A virus infection

HAV is a small positive-strand RNA virus that is shed in feces as naked nonenveloped virions [2]. Consequently, this virus is characterized by a high resistance in the environment and is primarily transmitted by the fecal-oral route, through direct contact with an infected person or ingestion of contaminated water or food [3].

This transmission explains the fact that the endemicity level of HAV infection, in a particular region in the world, is closely related to socioeconomic indicators and standards of hygiene and sanitation, especially access to clean drinking water. Serological prevalence surveys, based on the detection of total anti-HAV antibodies in serum samples at different ages, are the most useful tool to assess the endemicity of HAV infection. Up to date, four levels of HAV endemicity are defined according to the World Health Organization (WHO) [3]: high (≥90% by age 10 years); intermediate (≥50% by age 15 years, with <90% by age 10 years); low (≥50% by age 30 years, with <50% by age 15); and very low (<50% by age 30 years).

The clinical expression of HAV infection is highly age-dependent, ranging from asymptomatic form, frequently observed in early childhood, to fulminant hepatitis which particularly occurs in older age groups with chronic liver disease [4]. In low-income areas, including sub-Saharan Africa and South Asia, which are characterized by a high level of endemicity, HAV infection is acquired in young children, the age at which infection is often entirely asymptomatic. Thus, in these regions, the burden of hepatitis A is relatively low, and outbreaks are not common [1, 3]. By contrast, in high-income areas, including the United States, Western Europe, and Japan, which are characterized by a very low-endemicity pattern, HAV mainly circulates among specific groups at risk such as men who have sex with men, travelers in highly endemic countries, and intravenous drug users, leading to occasional relatively limited outbreaks [4]. Importantly, in many regions of the world, which are experiencing a deep change in HAV epidemiology such as some parts of Latin America, the Middle East, and Eastern Europe, large-scale community outbreaks are commonly observed. Indeed, improvements in socioeconomic status and hygienic conditions have led to an increase in average age at the time of infection, with adolescents and young adults being the predominant susceptible population, resulting in more symptomatic disease and therefore the occurrence of large epidemics in the community. These hepatitis A epidemics are often very difficult to control and represent a huge public health problem in these countries because of an increase in the incidence of severe illnesses, hospitalizations, and deaths related to this infection. These observations suggest what is known as "the epidemiological transition or shift" [1], which means that the decrease in HAV transmission rate is paradoxically associated to an increase in the incidence of symptomatic hepatitis A.

In Tunisia, HAV infection is still common, but its epidemiology is undergoing a gradual shift. Indeed, improvements in hygiene and socioeconomic conditions have led to changes in the pattern of the age-specific seroprevalence of anti-HAV antibodies; specifically, the prevalence of anti-HAV antibodies in the age group under 10 years declined from 91% in the 1980s [5] to 44% in 2001 [6]. These results suggest that HAV transmission is decreasing among younger children, leading to the occurrence of a larger number of symptomatic cases among adolescents and adults and even more frequent large outbreaks. During the years 2007–2010, community-wide outbreaks of hepatitis A have been recorded in Sfax Governorate (center east of Tunisia), with the occurrence of severe forms [7]. The increase in the incidence of hepatitis A cases involved nearly all regions of the governorate, including urban and rural areas. During this period, well-delimited outbreaks were observed, especially household and primary school epidemics.

The annual and monthly distribution of hepatitis A cases from 2000 to 2011 showed an endemic circulation of HAV with an increase in the incidence of the disease during the fall and winter season [7]. Importantly, this distribution highlighted similar waves of large outbreaks during 2002–2005, in comparison with those of 2007–2010, suggesting the cyclical trend of HAV infection in Tunisia. The regular evolution of hepatitis A is typical of HAV epidemiological shift; the delay in the exposure to the virus has generated a huge number of susceptible adolescents and adults and significantly increased the average age at infection. As the severity of disease increases with age, this has led to outbreaks of hepatitis A [4]. Consequently, nearly all population will be immunized against HAV until growing cohorts of susceptible young people become predominant after several years, hence leading to new outbreaks.

Among the patients diagnosed during 2007–2010 [7], 35 and 33% belonged to age groups 6–10 years and 11–15 years, respectively, which confirms that susceptibility to HAV is shifting from early age to older children and even adolescents and young adults. However, this shift was more prominent in urban areas than rural ones since the mean age of patients in these regions was 14.8 and 8.5 years, respectively. Two primary school epidemics were reported in rural settings, as well as several household outbreaks. Epidemiological investigation in this study suggested that rural outbreaks may be related to a common source contamination of water. By contrast, in urban areas, the situation was quite different from that observed in rural ones, since the epidemic consisted of many sporadic small outbreaks with no epidemiological link found between HAV confirmed cases.

Indeed, in countries with HAV epidemiological transition, different endemicity patterns simultaneously exist due to differences in socioeconomic development and hygienic practices between regions [1]. Urban areas may benefit the most from improvements in sanitary conditions, especially access to improved water sources and improvements in sewage treatment methods, hence increasing the risk of large outbreaks among adolescents and adults. The heterogeneity in HAV endemicity patterns between rural and urban areas is typical of HAV epidemiological shift.

3. Molecular epidemiology of hepatitis A virus infection

HAV has a single-stranded positive-sense RNA genome of 7.5 kilobases (kb) long [2]. The viral genome has a single open reading frame (ORF), divided into three functional regions, designated P1, P2, and P3. The P1 region encodes capsid polypeptides (VP1, VP2, VP3, and a putative VP4), whereas the P2 and P3 regions encode nonstructural proteins associated with viral replication [8]. Six HAV genotypes are up to now identified; three genotypes (I, II, and III) are of human origin, and three (IV, V, and VI) are of simian origin [8]. When these genotypes are defined by sequence variation within the VP1/P2A junction, there is 15% nucleotide variation between genotypes and 7–7.5% nucleotide variation between subgenotypes. Despite genetic heterogeneity at the nucleotide level, only a single serotype of HAV exists [9].

Although HAV is primarily shed in feces, there is a strong viremic phase during infection which has allowed easy access to virus isolates and the use of molecular markers to determine their genetic relatedness [9]. Currently, molecular epidemiological investigations are widely performed and are considered as a very useful tool for the identification of HAV transmission patterns and the potential source of the water or food-borne hepatitis A outbreaks. A molecular investigation approach is primarily based on the determination of viral genotype and the genetic relatedness between HAV strains.

Up to date, few investigations on the molecular epidemiology have been performed in Tunisia. In order to characterize HAV strains during the large outbreaks occurred in Sfax, Tunisia, during 2007–2010 [7], a molecular epidemiological study was carried out [10]. Amplification of VP1/2A region of HAV RNA by nested RT-PCR was performed on the serum samples for 159 patients with available epidemiological information [7]. HAV RNA was detected in 80.5% of cases. No relationship was documented between the positivity of HAV RNA and both age and sex ($p = 0.179$ and 0.553, respectively). For HAV RNA-negative cases, the mean delay between onset of symptoms and sampling was 25.5 days (range, 5–47 days), whereas for HAV RNA-positive cases, this delay was significantly lower, with a mean of 10.2 days (range, 1–49 days, $p < 0.001$). These findings suggest, as previously described, that the positivity of HAV RNA is correlated to the sampling time [11–13]. This result can be explained by the short duration of viremia, during natural history of HAV infection. Indeed, viral RNA could be detected on an average of 18 ± 14 days following the onset of clinical symptoms [14]. Another reason for the negativity of HAV RNA is the storage conditions of serum samples (the optimal temperature for the storage of RNAs is −80°C), leading to the degradation of the viral RNA and consequently to the negativity of PCR.

Nucleotide sequencing was performed for positive samples by RT-PCR. Strain genotyping was carried out by the phylogenetic analysis of a 394-nucleotide fragment, encompassing the VP1/2A junction (from nucleotide 2896 to nucleotide 3289, according to HAV strain HM175). Phylogenetic tree was constructed with MEGA software version 6.05, by using Kimura's two-parameter model, with the neighbor-joining algorithm (**Figure 1**). The reliability of the tree was tested by bootstrap resampling of 1000 replications. Nine reference sequences were included in the phylogenetic tree. Nucleotide identity percentages were computed, using the p-distance model included in the MEGA software (**Table 1**).

All clinical HAV strains from different regions of Sfax Governorate belonged to genotype IA [10]. This result is in an agreement with those of other Tunisian studies, which demonstrated that the predominant genotype still continues to be IA [15–17]. In addition, HAV sequences were closer to GBM reference strain (isolated in Germany) than to Asian sequences, suggesting a close genetic relatedness with HAV strains isolated in Mediterranean countries. This concept of related HAV strains according to geographical origin has been previously mentioned in China [18]. Indeed, Asian HAV strains were closer to each other than to the other reported sequences in the United States and Germany.

The mean identity percentage between HAV sequences was 98.1% indicating that clinical HAV strains isolated during 2007–2010 outbreaks were closely related, which confirms the endemic circulation of HAV in Sfax. Nevertheless, phylogenetic analysis evidenced the presence of genetic heterogeneity among HAV strains and identified three different clusters; rural strains clustered together with high bootstrap value (regardless of the outbreak period), suggesting the highly endemic circulation of the same HAV strains in these settings. This close genetic relatedness is most likely related to a common source of contamination [18–20]. Interestingly, the majority of HAV strains isolated during school epidemics shared 100% sequence identity. Of note, the abrupt increase in the number of jaundiced persons, in rural schools, has occurred within a short period of time in two geographically distant settings (Sidi Abdelkefi and Menzel Chaker (Bir Mallouli)). This transmission pattern strongly suggests the presence of a single source for school outbreaks [8].

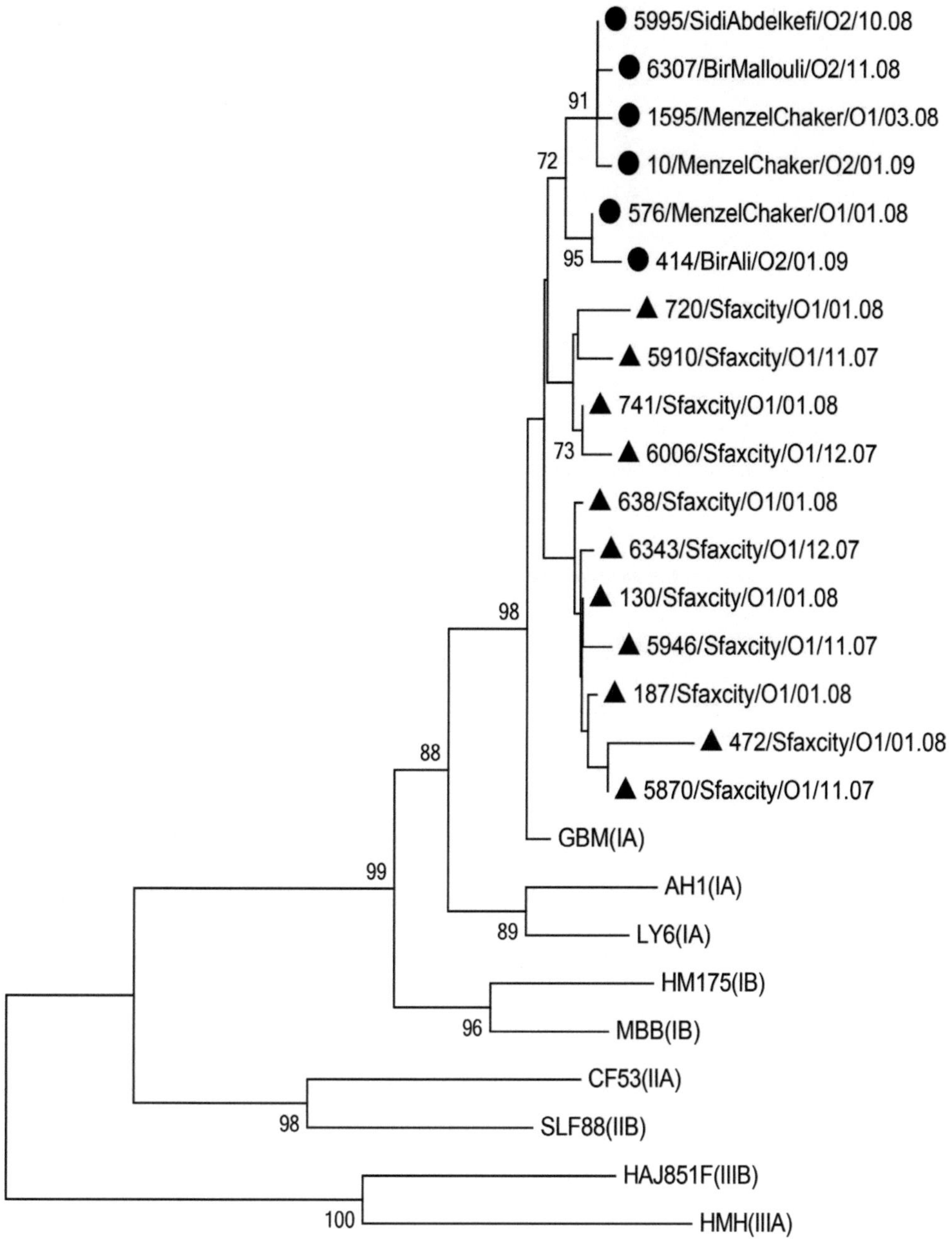

Figure 1.
Phylogenetic tree analysis of VP1/2A junction (394 bp) of HAV genome using Kimura's two-parameter model with the neighbor-joining algorithm. Numbers at tree nodes show bootstrap percentages obtained from 1000 resamplings. Bootstrap values <70% are hidden. Bars indicate genetic distances. Genotypes are shown in parentheses for HAV reference strains (see ***Table 1****). The Tunisian sequences are designated by their lab code followed by their region of origin, outbreak period (O, outbreak), and month and year of isolation. Sequences marked with a black circle indicate HAV strains recovered from rural areas, whereas those marked with a black triangle indicate HAV strains recovered from urban areas. For strains sharing 100% sequence identity, only one representative strain was included in the phylogenetic tree.*

Indeed, the epidemiological investigation highlighted the use by inhabitants of the same source of drinking water (private well) [7]. Inadequate sanitation, evidenced by fecal contamination of drinking water, in addition to the poor hygiene conditions indicates that the mainly route of HAV contamination is water transmission.

	Clinical sequences	
	% Nucleotide identity[a]	(Mean ± SD)[b]
Reference sequences		
GBM (IA)	96.9–98.7	
AH1 (IA)	92.8–94.3	(95.3 ± 0.7)
LY6 (IA)	93.3–94.9	
HM175 (IB)	90.7–92.3	
MBB (IB)	91.5–93.3	(92.3 ± 1.1)
CF53 (IIA)	84.3–86.1	(85.5 ± 1.5)
SLF88 (IIB)	84.3–86.4	
HMH (IIIA)	78.1–80.5	(80.3 ± 1.8)
HAJ85-1F (IIIB)	79.4–81.5	

[a]*Computed using the p-distance model included in the MEGA software.*
[b]*SD: Standard Deviation.*

Table 1.
Nucleotide identity between clinical and reference HAV strains.

Nevertheless, in these rural settings, interhuman transmission of HAV may also play a major role in the endemic circulation of the virus. In closed institutions such as schools, the agglomeration of individuals, sharing of objects, inadequate hygienic conditions, and high proportion of individuals susceptible to hepatitis A facilitate transmission [8].

HAV strains isolated in urban areas showed more genetic variability, since they were grouped into two different clusters, suggesting that urban outbreak may have originated from more than one source. In Sfax city, the epidemic consisted of many sporadic small outbreaks, which made it difficult to carry out a field investigation; thus, the information got from patients might not represent the whole situation in this large area. The genetic diversity of HAV strains was also reported in other regions in the world, where hepatitis A outbreaks observed in urban settings of industrialized countries cannot be linked to one source of contamination [18, 21]. The changing epidemiological pattern in HAV infection throughout Tunisia, particularly in urban areas, may result in more clinical cases in adolescents and adults and greater potential for new outbreaks. This changing pattern seems to be mainly related to improvements in hygiene conditions, since this study confirmed that genotype IA is widely circulating in Tunisia [10]. Thus, urban outbreaks are not linked to the other genotype emerging strains as it was reported by a Korean study [22], which showed that genotype IIIA becomes more prevalent than previously reported and may be the reason for the HAV outbreaks reported in Korea. Nevertheless, the higher genetic variability among HAV strains isolated in urban areas compared to rural ones in Sfax needs to be more evaluated by further molecular studies, in order to increase the understanding of hepatitis A epidemiology in these particular regions.

During urban outbreak, two fulminant hepatitis A cases were reported with fatal outcome, in one case due to an acute liver failure [7]. Unfortunately, only HAV strain from one patient was isolated. Since the time course between onset of symptoms and blood sample collection was very long (47 days), this could possibly explain the disappearance of viremia. It was previously suggested that viral determinants, in addition to host factors, could be involved in HAV disease severity, especially 5'UTR and 2B and 2C nucleotide substitutions [23, 24]. However, no correlation was found between HAV genotype and the different clinical outcomes [25].

Indeed, HAV strain recovered from one patient had 100% sequence identity with two other strains from patients with self-limited acute hepatitis A, indicating that infection with identical HAV strains within VP1/2A junction can result in drastically different clinical outcomes [8].

4. Conclusions

The findings of HAV molecular epidemiology study carried out in both rural and urban settings during large outbreaks in Sfax, Tunisia, in 2007–2010 strongly suggest that HAV infection is still highly endemic in rural settings, mainly related to the use of untreated water from contaminated sources, in addition to person-to-person transmission. However, genetic HAV diversity reported in urban areas, in comparison with rural ones, may reflect the epidemiological shift in these settings. Therefore, a close monitor of molecular HAV epidemiology is needed for a better understanding of HAV epidemiology in Tunisia.

Acknowledgements

The authors thank Mrs. Houda Abdelmoula for the English proofreading of this chapter.

Conflict of interest

The authors declare no conflict of interest.

Author details

Saba Gargouri[1*], Lamia Fki-Berrajah[1], Imen Ayadi[2], Amel Chtourou[1], Adnene Hammami[1] and Héla Karray-Hakim[1]

1 Laboratory of Microbiology, Habib Bourguiba University-Hospital, Faculty of Medicine, University of Sfax, Sfax, Tunisia

2 Laboratory of Molecular and Cellular Screening Processes, Centre of Biotechnology of Sfax, Sfax, Tunisia

*Address all correspondence to: sabagargouri@yahoo.fr

References

[1] Aggarwal R, Goel A. Hepatitis A: Epidemiology in resource-poor countries. Current Opinion in Infectious Diseases. 2015;**28**:488-496. DOI: 10.1097/QCO.0000000000000188

[2] Lemon SM, Ott JJ, Van Damme P, et al. Type a viral hepatitis: A summary and update on the molecular virology, epidemiology, pathogenesis and prevention. Journal of Hepatology. 2018;**68**(1):167-184. DOI: 10.1016/j.jhep.2017.08.034

[3] WHO position paper on hepatitis A vaccines-June 2012. Weekly Epidemiological Record. 2012;**87**(28/29):261-276. Available from: http://www.who.int/wer/2012/wer8728_29.pdf

[4] Franco E, Meleleo C, Serino L, et al. Hepatitis A: Epidemiology and prevention in developing countries. World Journal of Hepatology. 2012;**4**: 68-73. DOI: 10.4254/wjh.v4.i3.68

[5] Slim A. Etude de l'hépatite virale A chez l'enfant tunisien [thesis]. Faculté de Médecine de Tunis; 1982

[6] Letaief A, Kaabia N, Gaha R, et al. Age-specific seroprevalence of hepatitis A among school children in Central Tunisia. The American Journal of Tropical Medicine and Hygiene. 2005;**73**:40-43

[7] Gargouri S, Fki Berrajah L, Ayadi I, et al. Epidemiological and clinical analysis of hepatitis virus a infections during three successive outbreaks in Sfax (Tunisia) between 2007 and 2010. Médecine et Santé Tropicales. 2016;**26**:159-164. DOI: 10.1684/mst.2015.0491

[8] Vaughan G, Goncalves Rossi LM, Forbi JC, et al. Hepatitis A virus: Host interactions, molecular epidemiology and evolution. Infection, Genetics and Evolution. 2014;**21**:227-243. DOI: 10.1016/j.meegid.2013.10.023

[9] Nainan OV, Xia G, Vaughan G, et al. Diagnosis of hepatitis A virus infection: A molecular approach. Clinical Microbiology Reviews. 2006;**19**:63-79. DOI: 10.1128/CMR.19.1.63-79.2006

[10] Gargouri S. Epidémiologie clinique et moléculaire de l'infection par le virus de l'hépatite A dans la région de Sfax de 2007 à 2009 [thesis]. Faculté de Médecine de Sfax; 2013

[11] Hussain Z, Husain SA, Almajhdi FN, et al. Immunological and molecular epidemiological characteristics of acute and fulminant viral hepatitis A. Virology Journal. 2011;**8**:254. DOI: 10.1186/1743-422X-8-254

[12] Nainan OV, Armstrong GL, Han X-H, et al. Hepatitis A molecular epidemiology in the United States, 1996-1997: Sources of infection and implications of vaccination policy. The Journal of Infectious Diseases. 2005;**191**:957-963. DOI: 10.1086/427992

[13] Villar LM, Morais LM, Aloise R, et al. Co-circulation of genotypes IA and IB of hepatitis A virus in Northeast Brazil. Brazilian Journal of Medical and Biological Research. 2006;**39**:873-881

[14] Fujiwara K, Yokosuka O, Ehata T, et al. Frequent detection of hepatitis A viral RNA in serum during the early convalescent phase of acute hepatitis A. Hepatology. 1997;**26**:1634-1639. DOI: 10.1053/jhep.1997.v26.pm0009398009

[15] Beji-Hamza A, Taffon S, Mhalla S, et al. Migration pattern of hepatitis A virus genotype IA in north-Central Tunisia. Virology Journal. 2015;**12**:17. DOI: 10.1186/s12985-015-0249-9

[16] Gharbi-Khelifi H, Abid NBS, Beji A, et al. Seroprevalence and molecular characterisation of human hepatitis A virus in serum samples of Tunisian patients with clinical symptoms of viral hepatitis. Indian Journal of Virology. 2012;**23**:29-35. DOI: 10.1007/s13337-012-0063-6

[17] Neffatti H, Lebraud P, Hottelet C, et al. Southern Tunisia: A still high endemicity area for hepatitis A. PLoS One. 2017;**12**:e0175887. DOI: 10.1371/journal.pone.0175887

[18] Cao J, Wang Y, Song H, et al. Hepatitis A outbreaks in China during 2006: Application of molecular epidemiology. Hepatology International. 2009;**3**:356-363. DOI: 10.1007/s12072-008-9116-8

[19] Hutin YJ, Pool V, Cramer EH, et al. A multistate, foodborne outbreak of hepatitis A. National Hepatitis A investigation team. The New England Journal of Medicine. 1999;**340**:595-602. DOI: 10.1056/NEJM199902253400802

[20] Sánchez G, Pintó RM, Vanaclocha H, et al. Molecular characterization of hepatitis A virus isolates from a transcontinental shellfish-borne outbreak. Journal of Clinical Microbiology. 2002;**40**:4148-4155

[21] Costa-Mattioli M, Monpoeho S, Schvoerer C, et al. Genetic analysis of hepatitis A virus outbreak in France confirms the co-circulation of subgenotypes Ia, Ib and reveals a new genetic lineage. Journal of Medical Virology. 2001;**65**:233-240

[22] Lee H, Jeong H, Yun H, et al. Genetic analysis of hepatitis A virus strains that induced epidemics in Korea during 2007-2009. Journal of Clinical Microbiology. 2012;**50**:1252-1257. DOI: 10.1128/JCM.01114-11

[23] Fujiwara K, Yokosuka O, Ehata T, et al. Association between severity of type A hepatitis and nucleotide variations in the 5′ non-translated region of hepatitis A virus RNA: Strains from fulminant hepatitis have fewer nucleotide substitutions. Gut. 2002;**51**:82-88. DOI: 10.1136/gut.51.1.82

[24] Fujiwara K, Kojima H, Yonemitsu Y, et al. Phylogenetic analysis of hepatitis A virus in sera from patients with hepatitis A of various severities. Liver International. 2009;**29**:838-845. DOI: 10.1111/j.1478-3231.2008.01919.x

[25] Hussain Z, Das BC, Husain SA, et al. Virological course of hepatitis A virus as determined by real time RT-PCR: Correlation with biochemical, immunological and genotypic profiles. World Journal of Gastroenterology. 2006;**12**:4683-4688

Section 2

Hepatitis A: From Laboratory to Clinics

Chapter 4

Applications of Animal Models in Researching Hepatitis A

Huafeng Lin, Aiping Min, Gang Li, Yan Lei Chang, Lei Shi and Dan Qiu

Abstract

Hepatitis diseases are remaining in the list of significant threats to human health. Human hepatitis viruses are basically classified into six major hepatotropic pathogens—hepatitis A virus (HAV), hepatitis B virus (HBV), hepatitis C virus (HCV), hepatitis D virus (HDV), hepatitis E virus (HEV), and hepatitis G virus (HGV). Among these different forms of hepatotropic viruses, HAV as the leading cause of acute viral hepatitis is characterized as a kind of tiny ribonucleic acid virus that is linked to atopic disease. As we know, animal models have been instrumental in promoting understanding of complex host-virus interactions and boosting the advancement of immune therapies. So far, animal models such as nonhuman primates (NHPs) have enabled scientists to mimic and study the pathogenicities and host immune responses for hepatitis A infection. With the exception of chimpanzees and marmosets, animals like mice, pigs, guinea pigs, and tree shrews can also be selected as alternative animal models infected with HAV under laboratory conditions. In order to gain a better insight into hepatitis A pathogenesis and relevant contents, this chapter is mainly focused on the research progress in animal models of hepatitis A, and discusses the merits and demerits of these alternative models.

Keywords: hepatitis A, infection experiments, animal models, virus hepatitis

1. Introduction

Various forms of viral hepatitis represent a world health concern and challenge, generating a considerable socio-economic burden. Of these, hepatitis A as a type of food-borne hepatitis is mainly endemic in developing regions with the condition of inadequate sanitation and hygiene, such as in parts of Africa, Asia, Eastern Europe, South America, and Middle East [1, 2]. With the improvement of public health, the incidence of HAV infections in China have been gradually reduced (published data from 1990 to 2017) [3]. Up to now, 1.5 million cases of hepatitis A virus (HAV) infections are reported worldwide [2], which indicated that hepatitis A remains a primary problem in hygiene and public health. Hepatitis A has a very similar clinical symptom compared to hepatitis E. Except for the severer pathological injuries of hepatitis E than that of hepatitis A, both of two are self-limiting diseases, do not lead to liver cirrhosis and liver cancer, and transmit via orofecal route and person-to-person contact [4]. Consequently, HAV-contaminated water, vegetables, fruits, blood products, and other foodstuffs, especially undercooked shellfish including clams, oysters, and mussels (**Figure 1**) [5, 6], are the major pathways of infections

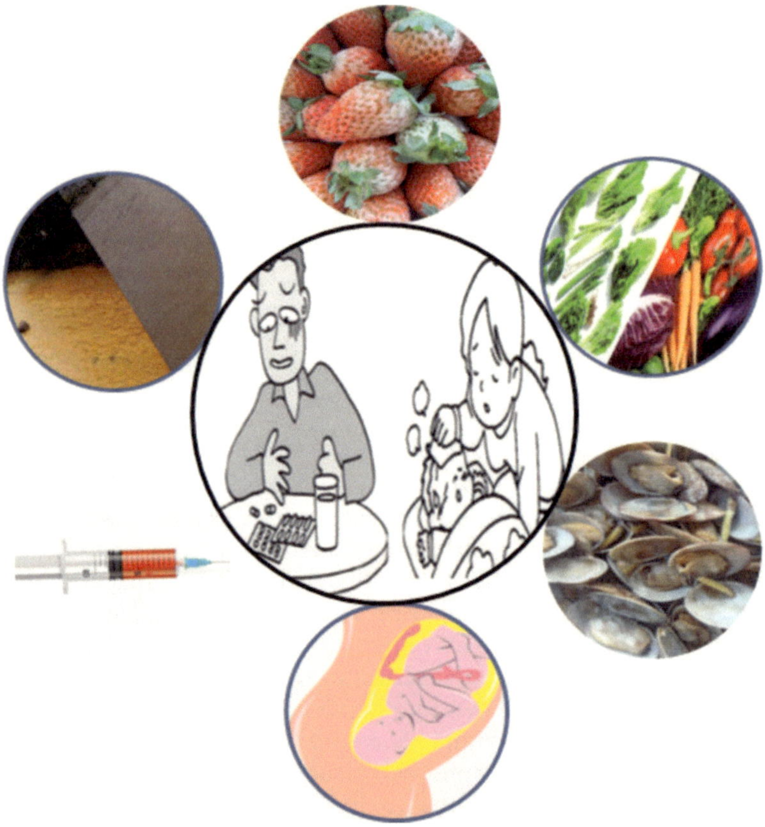

Figure 1.
Diagram showing the possible transmission routes of HAV.

with hepatitis A [7, 8]. Under certain circumstances, intravenous drug users with the collective use of syringes are at risk categories for HAV infections [9], and also there exist vertical transmissions of HAV from mother to child but occur very rarely (**Figure 1**) [10]. HAV as the main pathogen causing acute viral hepatitis is classified as a sole member of the genus Hepatovirus of the family *Picornaviridae*, which includes many medical and veterinary pathogens in 1991 [11–13]. HAV is a single linear positive-stranded RNA virus whose genomic full length is approximately 7500 nucleotides, which contain 5′-noncoding region (UTR), protein coding region, and 3′-noncoding region (UTR) (**Figure 2**) [13]. Researchers have found that HAV present in the form of naked, nonenveloped virions in feces aids to the viral transmissions through the environment. However, when HAV emerges in the blood of infected persons, the virion isolates itself from neutralizing antibodies by the way of producing quasi-envelope in host-derived membranes [14]. Epidemiological data showed that the most susceptible populations of HAV are the children in early childhood [2], and the disease prevalence exceeds 90% before the age of 10 [15], albeit most of infected youngers are usually mild or asymptomatic [16]. Hence, accelerating the immunological research and viral vaccine development can improve human immunity and reduce the spread of HAV. World Health Organization (WHO) recommends that vaccination combating HAV be integrated into the national immunization schedule for children aged ≥1 year on the consideration of many factors including cost-effectiveness [17]. What is noteworthiness is that, the illness infected with HAV in those people who are older than 60 will be very severe [18]. Moreover, HAV superinfections in chronic liver disease (CLD)

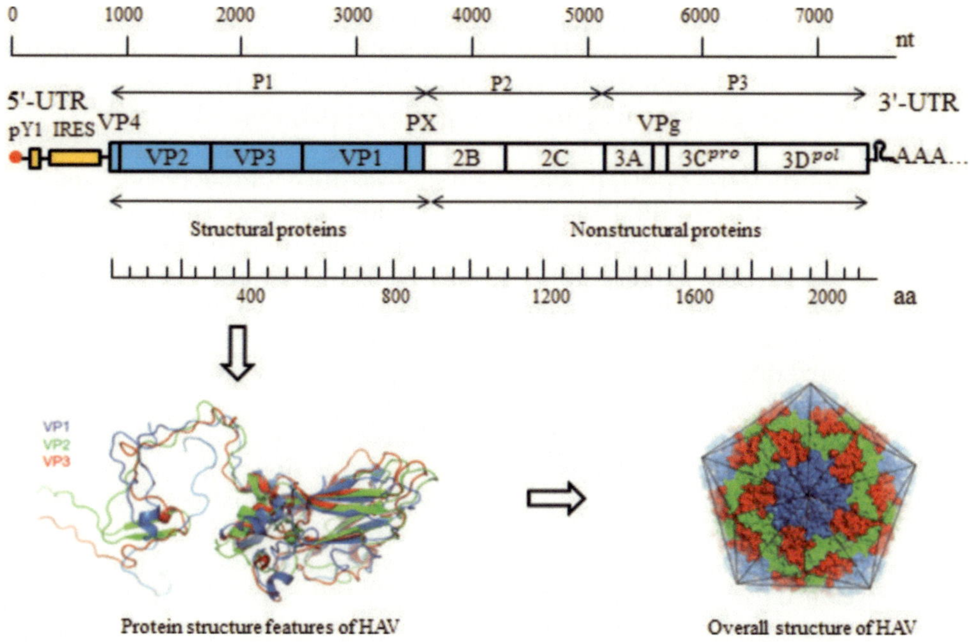

Figure 2.
The genome structure, protein structure components and overall structure of HAV. Refer to [28, 35, 36].

sufferers (e.g., hepatitis B or C) are usually associated with raising morbidity and mortality [19, 20]. To date, animal model is one of the promising tools in the investigation of human HAV infections. Studies on HAV immunopathological mechanism and host immune response mainly used nonhuman primates such as chimpanzees and marmosets as animal models. Due to the lack of other alternative animal models that support HAV infections, the study of the HAV biology and further development of therapies for hepatitis A have been hampered. Here in this chapter, the biological features of HAV will be discussed, the animal models of hepatitis A and their characteristics will be sketched, and the merits and demerits for these models will be analyzed as well.

2. Basic biological features of HAV and beyond

As early as 5000 years ago, hepatitis A-like illnesses were documented in ancient China. In Europe, similar disease known as "benign epidemic jaundice" was also described during the Hippocratic era [21]. As time goes by, in 1947, McCallum et al. termed infectious hepatitis as hepatitis A [22]. In the first half of 1967, Krugman et al. found the distinctive features between infectious hepatitis (hepatitis A) and serum hepatitis (hepatitis B) in clinical, epidemiological, and immunological aspects [23]. By 1973, Feinslone et al. firstly detected hepatitis A in feces of patients using the technology of immune electron microscopy (IEM) [24]. Morphologically and structurally, the purified HAV virion, having an outer diameter of 27–80 nm, is an icosahedral nucleocapsid protein granular which contains one linear positive-stranded ribonucleic acid (RNA) genome [25]. The genome encodes a single large polyprotein of 2227 amino acids [26], which is matured and folded to produce 10 biologically active viral proteins, including four structural proteins that construct the capsid (VP4 (~2.5 kDa), VP2 (24–30 kDa), VP3 (21–28 kDa), and VP1pX) and 6 nonstructural proteins that are indispensable for replication of the RNA genome (2B, 2C, 3A, 3B [VPg], $3C^{pro}$ [a cysteine protease], and $3D^{pol}$) (RNA-dependent

RNA polymerase) (**Figure 2**) [27]. By using standard serological technique and molecular identification methods, HAV is identified to belong to merely one single serotype, and is divided into seven distinct genotypes of which three genotypes (I, II, and VII) that circulate in humans, one genotype (III) isolated from either humans or owl monkeys, and other three genotypes (V–VII) exist in nonhuman primates [28–30]. Genotypes I, II, and III are sub-classified into subtypes A and B (Genotypes IA, IB, IIA, IIB, IIIA, and IIIB) [31]. Molecular epidemiology has further revealed that HAV sub-genotype IA is responsible for the most circulations among human population [32]. For sub-genotype IB HAV strains, several reports have declared that they were associated with food such as frozen strawberries in Australia and several countries of Europe [33, 34]. Recent studies of X-ray analysis have uncovered that HAV possesses a primitive capsid architecture related to that of picorna-like viruses infecting insects, which imply a correlation of primeval evolution as well as a novel cellular entrance mechanism for viruses [35]. The structure information (especially the 3D microstructural study) of viral protein is now a robust tool for dissecting their biological functions. In 2018, Stuart et al. reviewed updated studies on the structural features of outer protein shell of HAV and proposed the future researching scopes including relevant structural elucidations of the enveloped particles, as well as the capture of intermediates in the state of assembly, attachment, and/or uncoating [36]. In terms of receptor binding mechanism, Wang et al. pointed out that using a receptor mimic mechanism for neutralization of infectivity may hold promise for the therapeutic intervention of hepatitis A [37]. With regard to the origin of human HAV, phylogenetic analyses show that, in the remote past, these ancient viruses have emerged in different host species, and ancestral state reconstructions indicate HAV is likely to have originated in rodents [38]. What's more, investigations should be fundamentally focused on therapeutic interventions and new creations of HAV vaccines as a result of hepatitis A vaccine is one of the most effective strategy for the treatment of hepatitis A [39]. To date, four inactivated monovalent HAV vaccines from different manufactures (Havrix®, Epaxal®, Avaxim®, and Vaqta®) have been commercially available to the global markets [40]. Other hepatitis A vaccines such as a Chinese live attenuated vaccine (H2 strain, Zhejiang Academy of Medical Sciences, Hangzhou, PR China) and a Vietnam one are just self-sufficient in domestic production [41]. HAV infections are still an important cause of morbidity and mortality in developed countries such as the United States [42], let alone other nations with poor sanitation. Therefore, the work of scientific research for hepatitis A vaccine is still certainly on the way.

3. Applications of animal models

According to literatures, HAV strains of wild type are quite difficult in propagating in vitro. When culturing in cell-conditioned medium, they show low growth rate characteristically, as well as have no apparent cytopathic effects [43]. Additionally, HAV has its own special life history: it primarily replicates in the hepatic tissue, is excreted in biliary system to reach the intestinal contents [44], and is mostly shed in the feces and soil [45], where the viruses may persist for an extended period of time [46, 47]. Consequently, it is significantly important for researchers to find the proper infected models that aim at the investigation of HAV. As Hirai-Yuki and his co-authors have ever pointed out that, it is essential to develop improved animal models for the deeper investigations of the molecular and cellular mechanisms associated virus-hepatocyte interactions within the distinctive environment of liver tissue of hosts [48]. Here are the examples of disease models for HAV infections showed in **Table 1**.

Authors/year	Animal models	Comments	Refs
Dienstag et al/1975	Chimpanzees	Provided evidence for the susceptibility of chimpanzees to HAV	[49]
Amado et al/2010	Cynomolgus monkeys	Cynomolgus monkey was confirmed as a suitable model to study HAV infection	[67]
LeDuc et al/1983	New World owl monkeys	Confirmed the susceptibility of New World owl monkey to HAV	[53]
Song et al/2016	Pigs	First experimental evidence to demonstrate human HAV strains can infect pigs	[76]
Hirai-Yuki et al/2016	Mice	Provided a new paradigm for viral pathogenesis in the liver	[83]
Hornei et al/2001	Guinea pigs	Useful for studying some aspects of HAV pathogenesis and for testing the safety of vaccines.	[88]
Zhan et al/1981	Tree shrews	HAV can replicate in tree shrews and are potential for candidate models for HAV infections	[97]
Anthony et al/2015	Harbor seals	Describe the discovery of an HAV-like virus in seals	[98]
Liu et al/2019	Pekin ducks	There are differences in the pathogenicity of different subtypes of DHAV in ducklings	[100]
Wen et al/2019	Ducks	Provided new insights into the genetics and pathogenesis of DHAV-3	[101]

Table 1.
Examples of disease models for HAV infections.

3.1 NHPs

Broadly speaking, NHPs resemble humans in anatomy, physiology, and pathology over any other animals, which make them to be considered as the principal models for diseases including HAV infections. Human HAV has successfully infected various species of NHPs, such as chimpanzees (*Pan troglodytes*) [49], common marmosets (*Callithrix jacchus*) [50, 51], Squirrel Monkeys (*Saimiri sciureus*) [52], New World owl monkeys (*Platyrrhines*) [53], African green monkeys (*Cercopithecus aethiops*) [54], owl monkey (*Aotus trivirgatus*) [55], brown macaques (*Macaca arctoides*) [56], stump-tailed monkey (*Macaca speciosa*) [57] and tamarins, etc. (**Table 1**), but the host range of this virus is still narrow [58], mainly limited to relatively few species. The most common animal models used in laboratories for interrogating HAV infection are mainly marmosets and chimpanzees, which are of scarce resources (Chimpanzees are so expensive that they are not widely available for research use) in most countries. In addition, experimental data indicated that more than 90% of wild chimpanzees carried anti-HAV antibodies [59], which made them less suitable for investigating HAV-infectious diseases, but chimpanzees reared in captivity are more susceptible to infect hepatitis A. Moreover, it is very difficult for laboratory technicians to feed and operate experimentally on these two animals in many situations. And quite importantly, ethical concerns have advocated the decreasing use of chimpanzees for invasive experiments of research [60].

Take chimpanzees for example, they are the candidate experimental subjects that are most closely related to humans genetically, and most probably to be simulative and predictive of human outcomes when used as disease models. In 1962, Deinhardt et al. launched the initial attemption experiment that used chimpanzees to be infected with HAV through inoculating viral materials (serum or feces), but the gained results could not provide conclusive evidences for the transmission of infective hepatitis from humans to chimpanzees [61]. Intriguingly, in 1963, Hillis presented biochemical and histologic evidences that promisingly proved chimpanzees as useful as experimental hosts for human hepatitis viruses [62, 63]. In the mid-1970s, results of most of numerous publishment, which attempt to spread hepatitis A to chimpanzees yielded negative or equivocal results [64]. By 1984, Tsiquaye et al. carried out a study on acute hepatitis A infection occurred in hepatitis B chimpanzee carriers, which showed that superinfection can significantly alter the parameters of HBV chronicity in chimpanzees [65]. The authors pointed out that further observations were needed to establish the degree of severity of concurrent infection of HBV carriers with HAV, since such changes may have implications in some countries where the proportion of HBV carriers is high plus hepatitis A is highly prevalent [65]. For the purpose to locate where does the HAV might duplicate in the body, in 1989, Cohen and his colleagues conducted a study of single chimpanzee involvement in experiment, and found a possible oropharyngeal site for viral replication due to the emergence of HAV in saliva and throat swabs [66]. Similarly, Amado and co-authors acquired an experimental result that salivary gland was an extrahepatic site for early HAV replication in cynomolgus monkeys [67]. In the following two decades, the investigators shifted the focus of animal models to other NHPs instead of chimpanzees either because of the high cost of chimpanzee research or because of the poor contribution of chimpanzee experiments for biomedical applications [68]. Until 2011, Lanford et al. utilized three chimpanzee models to study the early innate immune responses to HAV infections. They found that HAV has a better property of keeping itself latent compared to HCV during early stage of acute resolving infection, and HAV infections represent a distinctly different paradigm in the course of intrahepatic interactions of virus-host [69].

The chimpanzees have been demonstrated to be an invaluable model tools for the investigation on HBV-induced disease pathogenesis and the discovery of novel prophylactic drugs and anti-viral therapies [70]. Optimistically, with the advancement of biotechnology, utilizing chimpanzee and other NHPs as disease models for HAV infection will surely play significant roles in HAV-associated studies in the future.

3.2 Pigs

Compared with NHPs, pigs have several advantages such as easy breeding and rearing, convenient handling and fewer ethical concerns, which make them be widely used in biomedical research [71]. Under natural conditions, it had been reported that HAV infections are being restricted to humans and nonhuman primates [72], and the appropriate models used for HAV infection have been restricted to nonhuman primates [73]. Due to several limitations of such animal models, other surrogate models need to be developed for further study. According to literatures, the immune system in pigs shares many similarities with humans for over 80% of analytical parameters, which made swine as a more suitable and common animal model for humans [74, 75]. Moreover, pigs have been used preclinically as disease models for preclinical studies usually. Until 2016, Song et al. firstly found the experiment evidence to prove human HAV strains can also infect swine [76], which took the first step to approach swine models for HAV infections. In this experiment, Song and colleagues observed that HAV can survive and replicate in pigs, which have replaced NHPs. However, there were no significant changes in the clinical manifestations and serum markers for pigs infected with HAV. Finally, they further suggested that pigs might be a suitable animal model for future studies related to HAV pathogenesis [76].

3.3 Chimeric mice/gene knock-out mice

Over the last two decades, mouse models have been successfully used in tackling various biological questions associated with intrahepatic immune response mechanisms for disease pathogenesis and clearing of HBV [77]. And also, such types of models can be applied to study the adaptive immune response to hepacivirus infection and will play roles in vaccine development. However, HAV is not capable to replicate in mice due to incompatibilities in the interaction of the virus and the innate immune system of mice. Therefore, scientists tackle this difficulty by utilizing chimeric mice, which facilitated the successful replication of HAV in the body through bypassing the cytosolic pattern recognition receptor, MAVS [78].

Generally speaking, certain cellular receptors are the key molecules that mediate viruses of entry into special kinds of cells in the body. Human membrane protein TIM-1 (T cell immunoglobulin and mucin domain protein-1) is a type of phosphatidylserine receptor that was firstly described as HAVCR1 [79], which helps cellular entry and infection with innumerable conventional enveloped viruses that bind phosphatidylserine on their surface [80]. And specially, TIM-3 receptor facilitates HAV for its entrance into target cells in humans [81]. However, recent research showed that TIM-1 is not an essential hepatovirus factor although its PtdSer-binding activity may contribute to the spread of quasi-enveloped virus and liver damage in mice [82]. For most of mouse models, wild-type mice are naturally resistant to HAV infection [83], and murine cell lines still exist defects in viral entry processes functionally [84]. For these reasons, multiple approaches have been developed by investigators to generate "humanize" mice at a genetic level to aid them susceptible to infection with HAV.

Previously, Yang et al. reported that, by using cell culture method, HAV ablates type 1 IFN responses thereby disrupting activation of IRF3 through the MDA5 pathway [85]. In 2013, Pang used HAV to infect SCID-beige/Alb-uPA mice with chimeric human/mouse livers for the purpose to test the susceptibility of mice to HAV. The result shows that these chimeric mice are permissive to HAV infection and represent valuable small animal models for future studies [86]. In 2016, Hirai-Yuki et al. applied the murine models with genetic defects in the induction of type I interferon (IFN) responses for HAV infection to reveal a previously undefined link between innate immune responses to virus infection and acute liver injury, which furnishes a novel paradigm for viral etiopathogenesis in the liver [83]. In 2018, a research team of Hirai-Yuki wrote a review of the study on "Murine models of hepatitis A virus infection" in which they provided an extensive and in-depth perspective into the development and application of mice models for HAV [48]. Additionally, in this chapter, it emphatically introduced the mechanism of degrading MAVS via viral proteases, in which it facilitates long-term survival of virus and spread through escaping from IFN-mediated restriction of virus replication and limiting pathogenesis and hepatic damage [48].

Till now, mouse models have been applied to support infections with HBV, HCV, and even HAV successfully. This probably has to do with building infections in the mouse liver, which is a key point in the development of viral hepatitis. Predictably, it has a promising future for utilizing mice as effective models for the investigation of HAV infection with the technological development of biomedical models.

3.4 Guinea pigs

The guinea pig models are more similar to humans than other small animal models in physiology and immunology. Specifically, the guinea pigs have the property of being analogous to humans in reproductive physiology and estrous cycle [87], etc. Guinea pigs have been used as an HAV infection model, but their use is limited because of the lack of development of anti-HAV antibodies in inoculated guinea pigs. In 2001, Hornei et al. conducted a study to determine whether HAV is capable to infect guinea pigs and whether they can be valid as a disease model for replicating HAV pathogenesis in humans and for the evaluation of vaccines [88]. The authors found that very low levels of HAV were detected in the livers of guinea pigs, which inoculated with human HAV [88]. Furthermore, they also described that the experimental guinea pigs shared similar response pattern with a New World nonhuman primate (*Callithrix jacchus*) after being challenged with HAV materials [88, 89]. The method of using guinea pigs to establish models for HAV infection is still under controversy. In 2010, de Castro Araujo and colleagues designed a research project to respond to the question "Whether HAV is capable to infect guinea pigs?". However, they failed to establish a guinea pig as model for HAV [90].

3.5 Tree shrews

Chinese tree shrew (*Tupaia belangeri chinensis*), mainly distributing in Yunnan and Guangxi provinces in China, is a class of small animals having a closer evolutionary relationship with humans compared to rodents [91]. Tree shrews have emerged in the vision of scientists for more than 30 years as a result of having many valuable features that are suitable in animals utilized as experimental models in biomedical studies [92], particularly in the fields of toxicology and virology [93]. To date, there are many attempts to employ tree shrews as models for human disorders such as hepatitis B [94] and hepatitis C infections [95, 96]. In 1981, Zhan et al. used fecal suspension of hepatitis A patients (concentration: 5%) to infect nine tree shrews through oral route, and eventually no apparent clinical symptoms of acute hepatitis were found. About 7–13 days after the viral infections, seven tree shrews were detected HAV that lies in their stools in 12–27 days, which indicated that HAV could reproduce in the body of tree shrews. The experimental results indicated that HAV can replicate in tree shrews and are potential for candidate models for HAV infections [97]. Additionally, they also found disease symptoms including increased alanine transaminase (ALT), hepatic hyperemia, hepatic edema, steatosis, and hyperplasia of Kupffer cells in the infected tree shrews, which further manifested that HAV can propagate in tree shrews [97].

3.6 Other animal models

Early studies suggested that HAV was unable to lead to infections of any common small laboratory animals successfully except NHPs. However, this "prejudice" has already been challenged and overturned by animal model engineering as well as by new scientific discoveries. In 2015, several strains of human HAV have been found in seals, which may indicate that the first natural nonprimate HAV to be discovered, and provide further understanding for the evolutionary history and pathogenicity of HAV [98]. Moreover, in recent years, HAV-associated hepatoviruses have been found in bats, rodents, hedgehogs [38], duck [99–101], and woodchucks [102, 103], which suggested that there may be more candidate animals potentially used as animal models of HAV. On the contrary, some scholars believed that these new viruses are substantially more divergent from each other and from human HAV (including simian HAV), which is in accordance with them being assigned to several additional species in taxonomy [78].

4. Ethical aspects

The animal experiments definitely play an important role in the development of life sciences and medical sciences. Therefore, ethical analysis concerning animal experiments is essential because it cannot completely avoid the use of animals [104] in the process of biomedicine and preclinical medicine research. Specially, NHPs act as the particularly valuable models for testing interventions against the Ebola and Marburg viruses in the field of studying of current infectious diseases, which can effectively objectively simulate human diseases via infections in these animals [105], and further contribute to the development of new protective and therapeutic vaccines. At a certain level, ethical issues become more important than scientific interest for this type of animal test [104] because such infections are often lethal to the experimental animals, which are commonly viewed as unethical. Similarly, experiments with HAV infection also expose animals (mainly NHPs) to injury or disease. Consequently, how to balance the contradiction between ethical challenges and NHPs infectious experiments becomes a vitally important subject.

5. Future directions

5.1 Animal model methods

Animal model research is entering a new and exciting stage along with the technologies of computational information and molecular biochemistry. For example, it is now possible for us to employ genome-edited techniques (e.g., ZFNs, TALENs, and CRISPR/Cas) to knockout specific genes, to knock in new genes, or to introduce specific mutations, and then to produce valuable animal models that benefited for our investigations. However, as we know, "no model is perfect, but many are useful" [106]. Therefore, establishing susceptible animal models is one of the methods in the research fields of HAV. By using appropriate and reliable animal models, virologist can perform a series of studies associated with hepatitis A including epidemiologic features, viral infectivity, humoral and cellular immunity, cytokine responses, virus pathogenesis, as well as the research and development of antiviral vaccinations.

5.2 Cell culture methods

For the development of hepatitis A vaccines, it is worth mentioning that a highly effective vaccine against HAV was manufactured by classical inactivation of the whole virus generated from cell culture [107], which commendably avoids the ethical controversy of using NHPs models. Moreover, there is a need to provide more support for the studies of long-term protection vaccines against hepatitis A infection [108].

Last but not least, it is very likely that a much wider host range of HAV-associated viruses will be discovered in other mammalian species in the future [38].

6. Conclusion

The Nobel laureate Peter Medawar have ever succinctly concluded that "No virus is known to do good" [109]. However, as we all know, "viruses are not omnipotent." For hepatitis viruses, the narrow hepatic tissue tropism maybe is the cause of constraining the host ranges of hepatitis viruses to relatively few special host species. As previously reported, only one serotype of HAV had been found globally [110]. However, according to Bosch et al., there exists the possibility of emergence of a novel serotype originated from zoonotic reservoirs [18]. In summary, it is necessary to further develop candidate animal models for hepatitis A infection although HAV is easily capable of adapting growth in the condition of conventional mammalian cell cultures [92].

In recent decades, HAV has been ignored by viral research circles to a certain extent due to the research spending and interest have shifted to other hepatotropic pathogens. Finally, animal model research, as a preclinical study aiming to hepatitis A, can offer a scientific platform to accelerate the pace for drugs screening and vaccines development.

Acknowledgements

We would like to express our sincere thanks to Professor Costin Teodor Streba, Professor Cristin Constantin Vere and Professor Ion Rogoveanu for initiating this book project.

Conflict of interest

No conflicts of interest were reported.

Financial support

This work was supported in part by grants from the National Key R&D Program Projects (2017YFF0104904), National Key Research and Development Plan (2016YFD0500600), Guangdong Provincial Science and Technology Plan Project (2017B020207004), Maternal and Child Health Molecular Genetic Medicine Research Project of Maternal and Child Health Center in Chinese CDCP (FY-ZX-ZD-0285, MHBD-0833-001), Youth Innovation Project of Sichuan Medical Research (Q16036), Key Science & Technology Project of Leshan in 2018 (18SZD150).

Acronyms and abbreviations

ALT	alanine transaminase
CLD	chronic liver disease
DHAV	duck hepatitis A virus
HAV	hepatitis A virus
HBV	hepatitis B virus
HCV	hepatitis C virus
HDV	hepatitis D virus
HEV	hepatitis E virus
HGV	hepatitis G virus
IEM	immune electron microscopy
IFN	type I interferon
IRES	internal ribosomal entry site
NHPs	nonhuman primates

TALENs	transcription activator-like effector nucleases
WHO	World Health Organization
ZFNs	zinc finger nucleases

Author details

Huafeng Lin[1,2†], Aiping Min[3*†], Gang Li[4†], Yan Lei Chang[2], Lei Shi[2] and Dan Qiu[5]

1 Department of Biotechnology, College of Life Science and Technology, Jinan University, Guangzhou, Guangdong, P.R. China

2 Institute of Food Safety and Nutrition, Jinan University, Guangzhou, P.R. China

3 Department of Gynecology and Obstetrics, The People's Hospital of Leshan, Leshan, Sichuan, P.R. China

4 Institute of Biomedicine and Department of Cell Biology, Jinan University, Guangzhou, Guangdong, P.R. China

5 Combined TCM and Western Medicine Clinics, College of Basic Medicine, Jinan University, Guangzhou, P.R. China

*Address all correspondence to: map5198@163.com

† These authors contributed equally to this work and should be considered co-first authors.

References

[1] Jacobsen KH, Wiersma ST. Hepatitis A virus seroprevalence by age and world region, 1990 and 2005. Vaccine. 2010;**28**(41):6653-6657. DOI: 10.1016/j.vaccine.2010.08.037

[2] Franco E, Meleleo C, Serino L, Sorbara D, Zaratti L. Hepatitis A: Epidemiology and prevention in developing countries. World Journal of Hepatology. 2012;**4**(3):68. DOI: 10.4254/wjh.v4.i3.68

[3] Sun XJ, Zhang GM, Zhou RJ, Zheng H, Miao N, Yin ZD, et al. Changes in the epidemiology of hepatitis A in three socio-economic regions of China, 1990-2017. Infectious Diseases of Poverty. 2019;**8**(1):1-8. DOI: 10.1186/s40249-019-0591-z

[4] Ren X, Wu P, Wang L, Geng M, Zeng L, Zhang J, et al. Changing epidemiology of hepatitis A and hepatitis E viruses in China, 1990-2014. Emerging Infectious Diseases. 2017;**23**(2):276. DOI: 10.3201/2302.161095

[5] Lap-Yee LAM. Detection of hepatitis A virus in shellfish in Hong Kong [thesis]. Hong Kong: The Chinese University of Hong Kong; 1998

[6] Hansman GS, Oka T, Li TC, Nishio O, Noda M, Takeda N. Detection of human enteric viruses in Japanese clams. Journal of Food Protection. 2008;**71**(8):1689-1695. DOI: 10.1002/jctb.1985

[7] Chaudhry SA, Koren G. Hepatitis A infection during pregnancy. Canadian Family Physician. 2015;**61**(11):963

[8] Acheson D, Fiore AE. Hepatitis A transmitted by food. Clinical Infectious Diseases. 2004;**38**(5):705-715. DOI: 10.1086/381671

[9] Hartard C, Gantzer C, Bronowicki JP, Schvoerer E. Emerging hepatitis E virus compared with hepatitis a virus: A new sanitary challenge. Reviews in Medical Virology. 2019;**29**:e2078. DOI: 10.1002/rmv.2078

[10] Shin EC, Jeong SH. Natural history, clinical manifestations, and pathogenesis of hepatitis A. Cold Spring Harbor Perspectives in Medicine. 2018;**8**(9):a031708. DOI: 10.1101/cshperspect.a031708

[11] Koff RS. Hepatitis A. Lancet. 1998;**351**(9116):1643-1649

[12] Vaughan G, Rossi LMG, Forbi JC, de Paula VS, Purdy MA, Xia G, et al. Hepatitis A virus: Host interactions, molecular epidemiology and evolution. Infection, Genetics and Evolution. 2014;**21**:227-243. DOI: 10.1016/j.meegid.2013.10.023

[13] McKnight KL, Lemon SM. Hepatitis A virus genome organization and replication strategy. Cold Spring Harbor Perspectives in Medicine. 2018;**8**(12):a033480. DOI: 10.1101/cshperspect.a033480

[14] Lemon SM, Walker CM. Hepatitis A virus and hepatitis E virus: Emerging and re-emerging enterically transmitted hepatitis viruses. Cold Spring Harbor Perspectives in Medicine. 2019;**9**(6):a031823. DOI: 10.1101/cshperspect.a031823

[15] Neffatti H, Lebraud P, Hottelet C, Gharbi J, Challouf T, Roque-Afonso AM. Southern Tunisia: A still high endemicity area for hepatitis A. PLoS One. 2017;**12**(4):e0175887. DOI: 10.1371/journal.pone.0175887

[16] Koff RS. Clinical manifestations and diagnosis of hepatitis A virus infection. Vaccine. 1992;**10**:S15-S17. DOI: 10.1016/0264-410X(92)90533-P

[17] World Health Organization. WHO position paper on hepatitis A vaccines.

Weekly Epidemiological Record. 2012;**87**(28-29):261-276

[18] Bosch A, Pintó RM, Guix S. Foodborne viruses. Current Opinion in Food Science. 2016;**8**:110-119. DOI: 10.1016/j.cofs.2016.04.002

[19] Vogt TM, Wise ME, Bell BP, Finelli L. Declining hepatitis A mortality in the United States during the era of hepatitis A vaccination. The Journal of Infectious Diseases. 2008;**197**(9):1282-1288. DOI: 10.1086/586899

[20] Debing Y. Towards the development of potent and selective inhibitors of hepatitis A and E virus [thesis]. Belgium: University of Leuven; 2015

[21] Feinstone SM. History of the discovery of hepatitis A virus. Cold Spring Harbor Perspectives in Medicine. 2019;**9**(5):a031740. DOI: 10.1101/cshperspect.a031740

[22] MacCallum FO. Homologous serum jaundice. Lancet. 1947;**250**(6480):691-692

[23] Krugman S, Giles JP, Hammond J. Infectious hepatitis: Evidence for two distinctive clinical, epidemiological, and immunological types of infection. JAMA. 1967;**200**(5):365-373. DOI: 10.1001/jama.1967.03120180053006

[24] Feinstone SM, Kapikian AZ, Purcell RH. Hepatitis A: Detection by immune electron microscopy of a viruslike antigen associated with acute illness. Science. 1973;**182**(4116):1026-1028. DOI: 10.1126/science.182.4116.1026

[25] Debing Y, Neyts J, Thibaut, HJ. Molecular biology and inhibitors of hepatitis A virus. Medicinal research reviews. 2014;**34**(5):895-917. DOI: 10.1002/med

[26] Yong HT, Son R. Hepatitis A virus: A general overview. International Food Research Journal. 2009;**16**:455-467

[27] Lemon SM, Ott JJ, Van Damme P, Shouval D. Type A viral hepatitis: A summary and update on the molecular virology, epidemiology, pathogenesis and prevention. Journal of Hepatology. 2018;**68**(1):167-184. DOI: 10.1016/j.jhep. 2017.08.034

[28] Walker CM, Feng Z, Lemon SM. Reassessing immune control of hepatitis A virus. Current Opinion in Virology. 2015;**11**:7-13. DOI: 10.1016/j.coviro.2015.01.003

[29] Robertson BH, Jansen RW, Khanna B, Totsuka A, Nainan OV, Siegl G, et al. Genetic relatedness of hepatitis A virus strains recovered from different geographical regions. Journal of General Virology. 1992;**73**(6):1365-1377. DOI: 10.1099/0022-1317-73-6-1365

[30] Costa-Mattioli M, Cristina J, Romero H, Perez-Bercof R, Casane D, Colina R, et al. Molecular evolution of hepatitis A virus: A new classification based on the complete VP1 protein. Journal of Virology. 2002;**76**(18):9516-9525. DOI: 10.1128/JVI.76.18.9516-9525.2002

[31] Cella E, Golkocheva-Markova EN, Trandeva-Bankova D, Gregori G, Bruni R, Taffon S, et al. The genetic diversity of hepatitis A genotype I in Bulgaria. Medicine. 2018;**97**(3):1-9. DOI: 10.1097/MD.0000000000009632

[32] FitzSimons D, Hendrickx G, Vorsters A, Van Damme P. Hepatitis A and E: Update on prevention and epidemiology. Vaccine. 2010;**28**(3):583-588. DOI: 10.1016/j.vaccine.2009.10.136

[33] Ruchusatsawat K, Wongpiyabovorn J, Kawidam C, Thiemsing L, Sangkitporn S, Yoshizaki S, et al. An outbreak of acute hepatitis caused by genotype IB hepatitis A viruses contaminating the water supply in Thailand. Intervirology. 2016;**59**(4):197-203. DOI: 10.1159/000455856

[34] Enkirch T, Eriksson R, Persson S, Schmid D, Aberle SW, Löf E, et al. Hepatitis A outbreak linked to imported frozen strawberries by sequencing, Sweden and Austria, June to September 2018. Eurosurveillance. 2018;**23**(41): 1-7. DOI: 10.2807/1560-7917. ES.2018.23.41.1800528

[35] Wang X, Ren J, Gao Q, Hu Z, Sun Y, Li X, et al. Hepatitis A virus and the origins of picornaviruses. Nature. 2015;**517**(7532):85. DOI: 10.1038/ nature13806

[36] Stuart DI, Ren J, Wang X, Rao Z, Fry EE. Hepatitis A virus capsid structure. Cold Spring Harbor Perspectives in Medicine. 2019;**9**(5):pii: a031807. DOI: 10.1101/cshperspect. a031807

[37] Wang X, Zhu L, Dang M, Hu Z, Gao Q, Yuan S, et al. Potent neutralization of hepatitis A virus reveals a receptor mimic mechanism and the receptor recognition site. Proceedings of the National Academy of Sciences. 2017;**114**(4):770-775. DOI: 10.1073/ pnas.1616502114

[38] Drexler JF, Corman VM, Lukashev AN, van den Brand JM, Gmyl AP, Bruenink S, et al. Evolutionary origins of hepatitis A virus in small mammals. Proceedings of the National Academy of Sciences. 2015;**112**(49):15190-15195. DOI: 10.1073/pnas.1516992112

[39] Liu XE, Chen HY, Liao Z, Zhou Y, Wen H, Peng S, et al. Comparison of immunogenicity between inactivated and live attenuated hepatitis A vaccines among young adults: A 3-year follow-up study. The Journal of Infectious Diseases. 2015;**212**(8):1232-1236. DOI: 10.1093/infdis/jiv213

[40] Chappuis F, Farinelli T, Deckx H, Sarnecki M, Go O, Salzgeber Y, et al. Immunogenicity and estimation of antibody persistence following vaccination with an inactivated virosomal hepatitis A vaccine in adults: A 20-year follow-up study. Vaccine. 2017;**35**(10):1448-1454. DOI: 10.1016/j. vaccine.2017.01.031

[41] Vesikari T, Van Damme P, editors. Pediatric Vaccines and Vaccination. Switzerland: Springer; 2017. p. 101. DOI: 10.1007/978-3-319-59952-6

[42] Hofmeister MG, Foster MA, Teshale EH. Epidemiology and transmission of hepatitis A virus and hepatitis E virus infections in the United States. Cold Spring Harbor Perspectives in Medicine. 2019;**9**(4):a033431. DOI: 10.1101/cshperspect. a033431

[43] Yokosuka O. Molecular biology of hepatitis A virus: Significance of various substitutions in the hepatitis A virus genome. Journal of Gastroenterology and Hepatology. 2000;**15**:91-97. DOI: 10.1046/j.1440-1746.2000.02141.x

[44] Hirai-Yuki A, Hensley L, Whitmire JK, Lemon SM. Biliary secretion of quasi-enveloped human hepatitis A virus. MBio. 2016;**7**(6):e01998-e01916. DOI: 10.1128/mBio.01998-16

[45] Wasley A, Fiore A, Bell BP. Hepatitis A in the era of vaccination. Epidemiologic Reviews. 2006;**28**(1):101-111. DOI: 10.1093/epirev/mxj012

[46] Siegl G, Weitz M, Kronauer G. Stability of hepatitis A virus. Intervirology. 1984;**22**(4):218-226. DOI: 10.1159/000149554

[47] McCaustland KA, Bond WW, Bradley DW, Ebert JW, Maynard JE. Survival of hepatitis A virus in feces after drying and storage for 1 month. Journal of Clinical Microbiology. 1982;**16**(5):957-958

[48] Hirai-Yuki A, Whitmire JK, Joyce M, Tyrrell DL, Lemon SM. Murine models of hepatitis A virus infection. Cold Spring Harbor Perspectives in Medicine.

2019;**9**(1):a031674. DOI: 10.1101/cshperspect.a031674

[49] Dienstag JL, Feinstone SM, Purcell RH, Hoofnagle JH, Barker LF, London WT, et al. Experimental infection of chimpanzees with hepatitis A virus. Journal of Infectious Diseases. 1975;**132**(5):532-545. DOI: 10.1093/infdis/132.5.532

[50] Mansfield K. Marmoset models commonly used in biomedical research. Comparative Medicine. 2003;**53**(4):383-392. DOI: 10.1053/svms.2003.YSVMS27

[51] Pinto MA, Marchevsky RS, Baptista ML, de Lima MA, Pelajo-Machado M, Vitral CL, et al. Experimental hepatitis A virus (HAV) infection in *Callithrix jacchus*: Early detection of HAV antigen and viral fate. Experimental and Toxicologic Pathology. 2002;**53**(6):413-420. DOI: 10.1078/0940-2993-00212

[52] Vitral CL, Yoshida CF, Marchevsky RS, Pinto MA, Teixeira CS, Baptista ML, et al. Studies on transmission of hepatitis A virus to squirrel monkeys. Primates. 2000;**41**(2):127-135. DOI: 10.1007/bf02557794

[53] LeDuc JW, Lemon SM, Keenan CM, Graham RR, Marchwicki RH, Binn LN. Experimental infection of the New World owl monkey (*Aotus trivirgatus*) with hepatitis A virus. Infection and Immunity. 1983;**40**(2):766-772

[54] Andzhaparidze AG, Balaian MS, Savinov AP, Kazachkov IUA, Titova IP. Spontaneous hepatitis similar to hepatitis A in African green monkeys. Voprosy Virusologii. 1987;**32**(6):681-686. DOI: 10.1016/0168-1702(87)90009-8

[55] Trahan CJ, Leduc JW, Staley EC, Binn LN, Bancroft WH. Induced oral infection of the owl monkey (aotus trivirgatus) with hepatitis A virus. Laboratory Animal Science. 1987;**37**(1):45-50. DOI: 10.1111/j.1748-5827.1987.tb05981.x

[56] Andzhaparidze AG, Shevtsov ZV, Korzaia LI, Karetnyĭ I, Balaian MS. Signs of natural infection with hepatitis A in brown macaques (*Macaca arctoides*). Voprosy Virusologii. 1987;**32**(5):541-544

[57] Mao JS, Go YY, Huang HY, Yu PH, Huang BZ, Ding ZS, et al. Susceptibility of monkeys to human hepatitis A virus. Journal of Infectious Diseases. 1981;**144**(1):55-60. DOI: 10.1093/infdis/144.1.55

[58] Lemon SM. Type A viral hepatitis: New developments in an old disease. New England Journal of Medicine. 1985;**313**(17):1059-1067. DOI: 10.1056/NEJM198510243131706

[59] Kessler H, Tsiquaye KN, Smith H, Jones DM, Zuckerman AJ. Hepatitis A and B at the London zoo. Journal of Infection. 1982;**4**(1):63-67. DOI: 10.1016/S0163-4453(82)91075-1

[60] Hutson S. Following Europe's lead, congress moves to ban ape research. Nature Medicine. 2010;**16**(10):1057. DOI: 10.1038/nm1010-1057a

[61] Deinhardt F, Courtois G, Dherte P, Osterrieth P, Ninane G, Henle G, et al. Studies of liver function tests in chimpanzees after inoculation with human infectious hepatitis virus. American Journal of Hygiene. 1962;**75**(3):311-321. DOI: 10.1371/journal.ppat.1003810

[62] Hillis WD. Viral hepatitis associated with sub-human primates. Transfusion. 1963;**3**(6):445-454. DOI: 10.1111/j.1537-2995.1963.tb04673.x

[63] Hillis WD. An outbreak of infectious hepatitis among chimpanzee handlers at a United States Air Force base. American Journal of Hygiene. 1963;**73**:316-328. DOI: 10.1093/oxfordjournals.aje.a120191

[64] Purcell RH, Emerson SU. Animal models of hepatitis A and E. ILAR Journal. 2001;**42**(2):161-177. DOI: 10.1093/ilar.42.2.161

[65] Tsiquaye KN, Harrison TJ, Portmann B, Hu S, Zuckerman AJ. Acute hepatitis A infection in hepatitis B chimpanzee carriers. Hepatology. 1984;**4**(3):504-509. DOI: 10.1002/hep.1840040325

[66] Cohen JI, Feinstone S, Purcell RH. Hepatitis A virus infection in a chimpanzee: Duration of viremia and detection of virus in saliva and throat swabs. Journal of Infectious Diseases. 1989;**160**(5):887-890. DOI: 10.1093/infdis/160.5.887

[67] Amado LA, Marchevsky RS, De Paula VS, Hooper C, Freire MDS, Gaspar AMC, et al. Experimental hepatitis A virus (HAV) infection in cynomolgus monkeys (*Macaca fascicularis*): Evidence of active extrahepatic site of HAV replication. International Journal of Experimental Pathology. 2010;**91**(1):87-97. DOI: 10.1111/j.1365-2613.2009.00699.x

[68] Knight A. The poor contribution of chimpanzee experiments to biomedical progress. Journal of Applied Animal Welfare Science. 2007;**10**(4):281-308. DOI: 10.1080/10888700701555501

[69] Lanford RE, Feng Z, Chavez D, Guerra B, Brasky KM, Zhou Y, et al. Acute hepatitis A virus infection is associated with a limited type I interferon response and persistence of intrahepatic viral RNA. Proceedings of the National Academy of Sciences. 2011;**108**(27):11223-11228. DOI: 10.1073/pnas.1101939108

[70] Wieland SF. The chimpanzee model for hepatitis B virus infection. Cold Spring Harbor Perspectives in Medicine. 2015;**5**(6):a021469. DOI: 10.1101/cshperspect. a021469

[71] Lin H, Deng Q, Li L, Shi L. Application and development of CRISPR/Cas9 Technology in pig Research. In: Chen Y-C, Chen S-J, editors. Gene Editing-Technologies and Applications. Rijeka, Croatia: IntechOpen; 2019. pp. 17-39. DOI: 10.5772/intechopen.85540

[72] Balayan MS. Natural hosts of hepatitis A virus. Vaccine. 1992;**10**:S27-S31. DOI: 10.1016/0264-410X(92)90537-T

[73] Lanford RE, Walker CM, Lemon SM. Nonhuman primate models of hepatitis A virus and hepatitis E virus infections. Cold Spring Harbor Perspectives in Medicine. 2019;**9**(2):a031815. DOI: 10.1101/cshperspect.a031815

[74] Zhao J, Lai L, Ji W, Zhou Q. Genome editing in large animals: current status and future prospects. National Science Review. 2019;**6**(3):402-420. DOI: 10.1093/nsr/nwz013

[75] Meurens F, Summerfield A, Nauwynck H, Saif L, Gerdts V. The pig: A model for human infectious diseases. Trends in Microbiology. 2012;**20**(1): 0-57. DOI: 10.1016/j.tim.2011.11.002

[76] Song YJ, Park WJ, Park BJ, Kwak SW, Kim YH, Lee JB, et al. Experimental evidence of hepatitis A virus infection in pigs. Journal of Medical Virology. 2016;**88**(4):631-638. DOI: 10.1002/jmv.24386

[77] Iannacone M, Guidotti LG. Mouse models of hepatitis B virus pathogenesis. Cold Spring Harbor Perspectives in Medicine. 2015;**5**(11):a021477. DOI: 10.1101/cshperspect.a021477

[78] Smith DB, Simmonds P. Classification and genomic diversity of enterically transmitted hepatitis viruses. Cold Spring Harbor Perspectives in Medicine. 2018;**8**(9):1-35. DOI: 10.1101/cshperspect.a031880

[79] Kaplan G, Totsuka A, Thompson P, Akatsuka T, Moritsugu Y, Feinstone SM.

Identification of a surface glycoprotein on African green monkey kidney cells as a receptor for hepatitis A virus. The EMBO Journal. 1996;**15**(16):4282-4296. DOI: 10.1002/j.1460-2075.1996.tb00803.x

[80] Moller-Tank S, Maury W. Phosphatidylserine receptors: Enhancers of enveloped virus entry and infection. Virology. 2014;**468**:565-580. DOI: 10.1016/j.virol.2014.09.009

[81] Sui L, Li N, Zhang W, Chen Y, Zheng Y, Wan T, et al. Human membrane protein Tim-3 facilitates hepatitis A virus entry into target cells. International Journal of Molecular Medicine. 2006;**17**(6):1093-1099. DOI: 10.3892/ijmm.17.6.1093

[82] Das A, Hirai-Yuki A, González-López O, Rhein B, Moller-Tank S, Brouillette R, et al. TIM1 (HAVCR1) is not essential for cellular entry of either quasi-enveloped or naked hepatitis A virions. MBio. 2017;**8**(5):e00969-e00917. DOI: 10.1128/mBio.00969-17

[83] Hirai-Yuki A, Hensley L, McGivern DR, González-López O, Das A, Feng H, et al. MAVS-dependent host species range and pathogenicity of human hepatitis A virus. Science. 2016;**353**(6307):1541-1545. DOI: 10.1126/science.aaf8325

[84] Asanaka M, Lai MM. Cell fusion studies identified multiple cellular factors involved in mouse hepatitis virus entry. Virology. 1993;**197**(2):732-741. DOI: 10.1006/viro.1993.1649

[85] Yang Y, Liang Y, Qu L, Chen Z, Yi M, Li K, et al. Disruption of innate immunity due to mitochondrial targeting of a picornaviral protease precursor. Proceedings of the National Academy of Sciences. 2007;**104**(17):7253-7258. DOI: 10.1073/pnas.0611506104

[86] Pang D. To HAV or not to HAV: Novel hepatitis A virus (HAV) infection in a chimeric mouse model [thesis]. Canada: University of Alberta; 2013. DOI: 10.7939/R3ZC7S536

[87] Kumar M, Krause KK, Azouz F, Nakano E, Nerurkar VR. A Guinea pig model of zika virus infection. Virology Journal. 2017;**14**(1):75. DOI: 10.1186/s12985-017-0750-4

[88] Hornei B, Kämmerer R, Moubayed P, Frings W, Gauss-Müller V, Dotzauer A. Experimental hepatitis A virus infection in Guinea pigs. Journal of Medical Virology. 2001;**64**(4):402-409. DOI: 10.1002/jmv.1065

[89] Baptista ML, Marchevsky RS, Oliveira AV, Yoshida CF, Schatzmayr HG. Histopathological and immunohistochemical studies of hepatitis A virus infection in marmoset *Callithrix jacchus*. Experimental and Toxicologic Pathology. 1993;**45**(1):7-13. DOI: 10.1016/S0940-2993(11)80439-2

[90] de Castro Araujo FR, Marchevsky RS, de Lima SMB, Martins LM, Hooper C, de Paula VS, et al. Guinea pig (*Cavia Porcellus*) can Be or not used as an experimental model to study hepatitis A virus infection? Virus Reviews & Research. 2010;**15**(1):1

[91] Chen M, Ou C, Yang C, Yang W, Qin Q, Jiang W, et al. A novel animal model of induced breast precancerous lesion in tree shrew. Biological and Pharmaceutical Bulletin. 2019;**42**(4):580-585. DOI: 10.1248/bpb.b18-00688

[92] Fan Y, Huang ZY, Cao CC, Chen CS, Chen YX, Fan DD, et al. Genome of the Chinese tree shrew. Nature Communications. 2013;**4**:1426. DOI: 10.1038/ncomms2416

[93] Fuchs E, Flügge G. Social stress in tree shrews: Effects on physiology, brain function, and behavior of subordinate individuals. Pharmacology Biochemistry and Behavior. 2002;**73**(1):247-258. DOI: 10.1016/s0091-3057(02)00795-5

[94] Yan RQ, Su JJ, Huang DR, Gan YC, Yang C, Huang GH. Human hepatitis B virus and hepatocellular carcinoma II. Experimental induction of hepatocellular carcinoma in tree shrews exposed to hepatitis B virus and aflatoxin B1. Journal of Cancer Research and Clinical Oncology. 1996;**122**(5):289-295. DOI: 10.1007/BF01261405

[95] Zhao X, Tang ZY, Klumpp B, Wolff-Vorbeck G, Barth H, Levy S, et al. Primary hepatocytes of Tupaia belangeri as a potential model for hepatitis C virus infection. The Journal of Clinical Investigation. 2002;**109**(2):221-232. DOI: 10.1172/JCI13011

[96] Feng Y, Feng YM, Lu C, Han Y, Liu L, Sun X, et al. Tree shrew, a potential animal model for hepatitis C, supports the infection and replication of HCV in vitro and in vivo. The Journal of General Virology. 2017;**98**(8):2069. DOI: 10.1099/jgv.0.000869

[97] Zhan MY, Liu CB, Li CM, Zhang WY, Zhu C, Pang QF, et al. A preliminary study of hepatitis a virus in Chinese Tupaia (author's transl). Acta Academiae Medicinae Sinicae. 1981;**3**(3):148-152

[98] Anthony SJ, Leger JS, Liang E, Hicks AL, Sanchez-Leon MD, Jain K, et al. Discovery of a novel hepatovirus (phopivirus of seals) related to human hepatitis A virus. MBio. 2015;**6**(4):e01180-e01115. DOI: 10.1128/mBio.01180-15

[99] Fu Y, Pan M, Wang X, Xu Y, Yang H, Zhang D. Molecular detection and typing of duck hepatitis A virus directly from clinical specimens. Veterinary Microbiology. 2008;**131**(3-4):247-257. DOI: 10.1016/j.vetmic.2008.03.011

[100] Liu R, Shi S, Huang Y, Chen Z, Chen C, Cheng L, et al. Comparative pathogenicity of different subtypes of duck hepatitis A virus in Pekin ducklings. Veterinary Microbiology. 2019;**228**:181-187. DOI: 10.1016/j.vetmic.2018.11.030

[101] Wen X, Guo J, Sun D, Wang M, Cao D, Cheng A, et al. Mutations in VP0 and 2C proteins of duck hepatitis A virus type 3 attenuate viral infection and virulence. Vaccine. 2019;**7**(3):111. DOI: 10.3390/vaccines7030111

[102] Yu JM, Li LL, Zhang CY, Lu S, Ao YY, Gao HC, et al. A novel hepatovirus identified in wild woodchuck Marmota himalayana. Scientific Reports. 2016;**6**:22361

[103] Sander AL, Corman VM, Lukashev AN, Drexler JF. Evolutionary origins of enteric hepatitis viruses. Cold Spring Harbor Perspectives in Medicine. 2018;**8**(12):a031690. DOI: 10.1101/cshperspect.a031690

[104] Gross D, Tolba RH. Ethics in animal-based research. European Surgical Research. 2015;**55**(1-2):43-57. DOI: 10.1159/000377721

[105] Barnhill A, Joffe S, Miller FG. The ethics of infection challenges in primates. Hastings Center Report. 2016;**46**(4):20-26. DOI: 10.1002/hast.580

[106] Baxter VK, Griffin DE. Animal models: No model is perfect, but many are useful. In: Viral Pathogenesis. New York: Academic Press; 2016. pp. 125-138. DOI:10.1016/B978-0-12-800964-2.00010-0

[107] Plotkin SA, Plotkin SL. The development of vaccines: How the past led to the future. Nature Reviews Microbiology. 2011;**9**(12):889-893. DOI: 10.1038/nrmicro2668

[108] Ott JJ, Irving G, Wiersma ST. Long-term protective effects of hepatitis A vaccines. A systematic review. Vaccine. 2012;**31**(1):3-11. DOI: 10.1016/j.vaccine.2012.04.104

[109] Cuthbert JA. Hepatitis A: Old and new. Clinical Microbiology Reviews. 2001;**14**(1):38-58. DOI: 10.1128/CMR.14.1.38-58.2001

[110] Seymour IJ, Appleton H. Foodborne viruses and fresh produce. Journal of Applied Microbiology. 2001;**91**(5):759-773. DOI: 10.1046/j.1365-2672.2001. 01427.x

Chapter 5

Hepatitis A: How We Are after the Introduction of Vaccines

Julia Teixeira Rodrigues, Priscila Menezes Ferri Liu and Adriana Teixeira Rodrigues

Abstract

Hepatitis A is a disease known for a long time. It has a universal distribution, although it has a higher prevalence in places with poor sanitary conditions due to its main form of transmission: fecal-oral. The local health conditions also influence the age of acquisition of the disease and, therefore, its clinical presentation, because the disease in young children is usually asymptomatic. It is a viral disease whose prevention is possible through improvements in the population's basic sanitation conditions and vaccination. Since the introduction of vaccines, it has been possible to see a reduction in its incidence, especially in places where universal vaccination of children has been instituted. In recent years immunoglobulin therapy is being replaced by vaccination in pre- and postexposure prophylaxis (PEP), except in specific situations. Its incidence, even in developing countries, has decreased after introduction of hepatitis A vaccine. The vaccine is recommended in two doses for children, starting at the age of 1. Argentina and, more recently, Brazil have adopted the universal vaccination of all children upon completion of 12 months of age in a single-dose regimen. Despite this breakthrough isolated outbreaks in homeless and drug users are still described in developed countries.

Keywords: hepatitis viruses, classification, diagnosis, prevention, control

Key points

- Hepatitis A is a viral disease whose prevention is possible through improvements in the population's basic sanitation conditions and vaccination.
- The incidence, even in developing countries, has been reduced since the introduction of vaccines against hepatitis A.
- The vaccine is recommended in two doses for children, starting at the age of 1.
- Argentina and, more recently, Brazil have adopted the universal vaccination of all children upon 12 months of age in a single-dose regimen.

While dealing with hepatitis A diagnosis, be aware of the signs of acute hepatic encephalopathy, because although it is a rare complication, it may require hepatic transplantation.

1. Introduction

Hepatitis A is an acute viral disease caused by the hepatitis A virus (HAV), a picornavirus that infects only primates and has a low mutation rate compared to the other viruses capable of causing acute viral hepatitis [1–3].

The hepatitis A virus is transmitted by the fecal-oral route, either through ingestion of contaminated food [1] and water [4] or person-to-person contact. It has the ability to survive on surfaces for up to 60 days, and it is relatively resistant to alcohol and ether. As a result, the hygiene of bathrooms and toys in day care facilities must be meticulous [2, 5, 6].

The disease endemic character is related to poor sanitation conditions. That explains why its prevalence is higher in developing countries, where children generally become infected during the first years of life. That justifies the predominance of the asymptomatic form of the disease in such places [2].

Although it is related to inadequate sanitation conditions, there are records of the disease even in developed countries where the major concern is the people, mainly adults, who travel to exotic locations or developing countries. Besides that, some outbreaks due to food contamination are also described. Adult's disease, unlike the one that occurs in children, is symptomatic in 80% of cases [2]. Fortunately, since the introduction of vaccines, there has been a progressive decrease in the number of the cases of hepatitis A [7].

2. The virus

Hepatitis A virus (HAV) is one of the five etiological agents of viral hepatic inflammation (HAV, HBV, HCV, HDV, and HEV), whose incidence, according to the WHO, is sporadic and occurs in the form of epidemics around the whole world, which tend to present cyclical recurrences [8]. It belongs to the genus *Hepatovirus* that belongs to the family *Picornaviridae* [9].

2.1 Structure of the virus

HAV is described as being a naked virus; however, there is evidence that it can be released from a preinfected cell, through a non-lytic path, inside a small extracellular vesicle whose membrane surrounds the entire capsid and provides protection against the mechanisms of the host immune system [10].

The HAV presents as a genetic material a single-strand RNA with positive polarity, which confers the ability to act as messenger RNA (mRNA) and to interact directly with the ribosome to initiate the synthesis of the viral proteins. Its genome is divided in three parts [11]:

1. Noncoding region 5′UTR covalently linked to viral protein VPg [11]

2. A single open reading frame (ORF) subdivided into P1, which encodes the viral capsid proteins (VP1, VP2, VP3, and VP4), and P2 and P3, which encode nonstructural proteins that act during viral multiplication [11]

3. Noncoding region 3′UTR which has a poly-A tail [11]

2.2 Biological cycle

The HAV is transmitted through fecal-oral route; the individual becomes infected from the ingestion of water and food contaminated by fecal material from another individual who had been previously infected.

After ingestion, the virus falls into the blood vessels and, through the portal circulation, reaches the hepatocytes. The first contact occurs through the basolateral membrane of the hepatocytes in the space of Disse [9]. After the processes of adsorption, penetration, denudation, and synthesis of viral genome and viral proteins, the virus is assembled and released from the host cell through a non-cytolytic process and undergoes cell exocytosis [12]. This release can occur through the apical membrane of the hepatocyte, which will cause the new virus to go to the bile canaliculi and, consequently, be sent to the intestine along with the bile. In addition, the release can also occur by the basolateral membrane, which causes the virus to return to the bloodstream [10, 12].

After being sent to the intestine, the virus will be sent to the external environment through the feces. During excretion, a large amount of virus is eliminated. This starts about 10 days before the onset of clinical manifestations [13]. The period of greatest transmissibility occurs between the previous 15 days and 7 days after the onset of symptoms [4].

3. Pathogenesis

The immune response built by the host leads to the destruction of the hepatocytes infected by the virus and causes the appearance of the symptoms and signs of the disease. The HAV's slow replication does not appear to cause cytopathic effects [13].

It is possible that several mechanisms are involved in the development of signs of the disease. In one study fibroblasts and peripheral blood lymphocytes from patients with acute hepatitis A were used to demonstrate that the IFN-γ produced by HAV-specific cytotoxic T lymphocytes might play an important role in the pathogenesis of the disease [14].

Another analysis evidenced the presence of IFN-γ, TNF, IL-2, and IL-21 produced by polyfunctional CD4 + T cells. These results place the immune response modulated by CD4 + T lymphocytes as being more crucial in the control of HAV replication [15].

In contrast to studies that propose that adaptive immunity is more important in the pathogenesis and resolution of hepatitis A, it has been proposed that cells of the innate immune system, especially natural killer and lymphokine-activated killer (LAK) cells, play a crucial role in hepatic cell damage, which is inflicted prior to that performed by cytotoxic T lymphocytes [16].

In addition, there is an antibody-mediated response. HAV-specific immunoglobulin M (IgM) antibody and IgA antibodies can be detected, from the onset of the first clinical signs, in the patient's serum or plasma during the acute phase of the disease. IgG antibodies appear 1 week after the onset of the disease and can be detected for years even after healing. IgG can also be detected in vaccinated individuals. IgM and IgG immunoglobulins can neutralize the virus by recognizing epitopes of the HAV's structural proteins, VP1, VP2, and VP3, located in the capsid [17].

4. Epidemiology

The hepatitis A virus is distributed worldwide. However, the highest incidence of hepatitis A occurs in developing countries and in the ones with poor health conditions. In developed countries the disease acquired by traveler accounts for almost half of the cases reported.

The introduction of universal vaccination of children can change this general picture. The implementation of this program may reduce the rate of seropositive children against hepatitis A virus [18].

Luxemburger and Dutta show Brazil as a country with high endemicity of hepatitis A, meaning that more than 90% of children between 5 and 14 years old were seropositive for hepatitis A [19].

After that date there have been modifications in epidemiology of this disease. Checking the Epidemiological Bulletin of the Ministry of Health of Brazil in 2018, it's possible to notice that after 2007 the incidence rate of hepatitis A has shown a progressive tendency of falling, going from 7.1 cases to 1.0 per 100,000 inhabitants in 2017.

Between 1997 and 2017, most cases of hepatitis A occurred in children under 10 years of age (53.8%). In the last 2 years, there has been not only an increase in the incidence of the disease among people from 20 to 39 years of age but also a modification in the route of contamination. There was a significant reduction in cases related to food contamination and an increase in those related to sexual transmission. The incidence reduction preceded the universal vaccine. Universal vaccination of children from 12 months onwards was introduced in Brazil's vaccination calendar only in 2014 [20].

In relation to hepatitis A mortality in Brazil, between 2000 and 2016, there were 1125 deaths associated with viral hepatitis A. There is no data yet to compare mortality after the onset of the universal vaccine of Brazilian children [20]. Considering the distribution of deaths associated with all viral hepatitis in Brazil between 2000 and 2016 (66,196 obits), the proportion of obits was 1.7% associated with viral hepatitis A; 21.4% to hepatitis B; 75.8% to hepatitis C; and 1.1% to hepatitis D. In the document there is no report of viral hepatitis E [20].

Recently, the person-to-person HAV outbreaks involving people who use drugs or people experiencing homelessness are ongoing in United States, and this could signal a shift in HAV infection epidemiology in the United States [21].

5. Clinical condition

The virus's incubation period is long (15–50 days), and the first symptoms are non-specific and reminiscent of common viral disease. The following may be present: fever, malaise, headache, and abdominal pain. Eventually, jaundice, hepatomegaly, splenomegaly, and bradycardia can appear. The icteric phase has a variable duration, on average from 4 to 30 days, and is associated with dark urine and acholic stools. Laboratory elevation of aminotransferases and direct hyperbilirubinemia is observed [2].

Hepatitis A can have different forms of evolution, although most patients progress to healing within 2 months. Approximately 10% of hepatitis A patients present a biphasic form, in which relapses are observed in the first 6 months of evolution. Other forms considered atypical [6] may also be observed as the prolonged form, in which the symptoms persist for up to 120 days [22], and the cholestatic form presents the following alterations: elevation of the direct fraction of bilirubin, presence of significant pruritus, malabsorption of nutrients, and weight loss. Fortunately, all these forms present evolution for healing. Only a small fraction of patients will develop acute liver failure that is associated with increased morbidity and mortality [22].

6. Diagnosis

According to CDC [23], suspected hepatitis A occurs in the presence of a suggestive clinical picture, characterized by the presence of fever, headache, malaise, anorexia, nausea, vomiting, diarrhea, abdominal pain, or dark urine, associated with suggestive laboratory alterations of the direct bilirubin fraction or ALT > 200 IU/L, in the absence of another diagnosis that explains such alterations.

The presence of immunoglobulin M (IgM) antibody against hepatitis A virus or viral RNA detection provides laboratory evidence for the diagnosis [23].

The presence of sensorineural alterations should raise the suspicion of acute liver failure, and the diagnosis is confirmed if there is an association of sensory alterations with a high prothrombin time in more than 4–6 s (INR $\geq$ 1.5) [24, 25].

7. Treatment

Hepatitis A has no specific treatment, and usually only support and monitoring measures are adopted. Although the disease is self-limiting in the vast majority of cases, some patients develop severe hepatitis, which can lead to fulminant hepatic insufficiency, and need liver transplantation.

The fulminant hepatic insufficiency diagnosis should be considered in those patients with viral hepatitis who present any alteration of consciousness accompanied by some coagulation disorder [23] characterized by INR $\geq$ 1.5. Those findings indicate hospitalization of the patient in an intensive care unit with possibility of transfer to a liver transplant center.

It is important to be aware of the fact that the symptoms of fulminant hepatic insufficiency become noticeable late when most of the liver functions are already compromised [26]. And so, the patient need to be transferred to a transplant center as soon as possible if he or she presents metabolic acidosis with arterial pH < 7.3, arterial lactate > 3 mmol/L (27 mg/dL), INR > 6.5, creatinine > 3.4 mg/dL, and presence of grade 3 or 4 hepatic encephalopathy all within the 24-h period [25].

Special attention should also be given to the child who evolves with the cholestatic form due to the nutritional risk secondary to malabsorption of fat-soluble nutrients and vitamins. During disease, until the cholestasis is fully treated, it may be necessary to provide increased caloric intake in addition to vitamins A, D, and E. Nutritional care should be maintained until cholestasis improves [27].

8. Prevention

The Brazilian Ministry of Health advices that the prevention of the disease is best achieved by improving basic sanitation and personal hygiene conditions as follows [28]:

1. Wash the hands after going to the bathroom and before eating or preparing food [28].

2. Wash, with treated water, foods that are consumed raw [28].

3. Cook the food before eating it [28].

4. Wash dishes, glasses, cutlery, and bottles properly [28].

5. Avoid the construction of ditches near wells and river springs, so as not to compromise the water table that feeds the well [28].

6. If there is a patient with hepatitis A at home, use 2.5% sodium hypochlorite, or bleach when washing the restroom [28].

7. In nurseries, preschools, cafeterias, restaurants, and closed institutions, adopt strict hygiene measures, such as disinfection of objects, benches, and floors using 2.5% sodium hypochlorite or bleach [28].

As a prophylactic measure for travelers, the vaccine has replaced immunoglobulin (Ig). The protection achieved by Ig when used before exposure is approximately 80–90% [20], whereas a single dose of hepatitis A vaccine provides protection of 85% of cases in the first 6 weeks and up to 95–00% after this time period [29]. Postexposure prophylaxis (PEP) with hepatitis A vaccine prevents hepatitis A virus infection when administered within 2 weeks of exposure [25, 30]. The use of Ig for PEP is indicated in the following situations: children aged <12 months; immunocompromised people; patients with chronic liver disease; and those for whom the vaccine is contraindicated. For people over 40, immunoglobulin is preferred, but the vaccine can be used on a non-distant immunoglobulin obtained [25, 28]. The recommended dose of IG was modified to 0.1 mL/kg [30].

Pre-exposure prevention for travelers aged 12 months to 40 years should be given by vaccination as soon as traveling to endemic sites is considered, and the second dose should be administered at the regular interval recommended by the vaccine manufacturer. The vaccine can be administered between 6 and 11 months for pre-exposure prophylaxis, but this dose should not be considered when the child initiates the usual vaccination schedule at 12 months of age. In the case of infants <6 months of age, Ig should be given. The dose in these cases depends on the duration of the trip: for trips with a duration of up to 1 month 0.1 mL/kg is recommended; and with longer duration, the dose will be 0.2 mL/kg repeated every 2 months until the end of the trip. Travelers aged >40 years, immunocompromised or with chronic liver disease, are recommended to be vaccinated against hepatitis A and use Ig at the dose of 0.1 mL/kg at the same time but applied at separate sites [30].

Since the introduction of vaccines, there has been a reduction in the prevalence of the disease. The vaccine is effective, even if given as a single dose, although it is usually recommended in two doses. The initial dose should be administered at 1 year of age, especially in endemic areas where contact with the virus is early. The booster dose may occur at varying intervals, usually 6–18 months after the first dose.

The effectiveness of the single-dose vaccine was initially described among people vaccinated for travel to exotic locations or with inadequate sanitary conditions [31, 32]. In 2003 a randomized, double blind study in Nicaragua showed that one dose of the vaccine had good efficacy, reaching up to 100% of children after 6 weeks (95% CI: 79.8–100%) [29].

Young children who present hepatitis A are asymptomatic and therefore able to spread the virus in the community. That is why universal vaccination of all children between 1 and 5 years of age is recommended in populations where the incidence of the disease is >20 cases/100,000 inhabitants. The monovalent vaccine (Havrix®, Vaqta®) should be administered via intramuscular injection in two doses at a 6- to 12-month interval between doses [21, 25].

In 2005, Argentina adopted a universal vaccination schedule for children aged 12 months in a single dose, and since then the incidence of hepatitis A has decreased by >80% in all age groups [33, 34].

For developing countries, this may be a cheaper and simpler strategy than two-dose schedules; however, it is necessary to deploy a surveillance system to determine in the long run whether the booster dose will be needed [34].

In Brazil, the hepatitis A vaccine was added to the national immunization program (NIP) only in 2014. Universal vaccination of children with a single dose of the inactivated vaccine was adopted at 12 months of age. In an official document, the NIP undertook to monitor the epidemiological situation of hepatitis A, aiming at the definition of whether or not to include a second dose in the child's immunization schedule [35].

The United Nations (UN) reports that viral hepatitis is a serious threat to global health, mainly related to hepatitis B and C viruses that cause chronic liver disease. The UN estimates suggest that 325 million people are infected worldwide, with 70 million on the African continent alone. Although the reports focus on hepatitis B and C because of their chronicity, the UN and WHO are committed to reducing hepatitis A-related deaths by 10 percent by the year 2030. According to the WHO, viral hepatitis A is a viral infection of the disease. It can be eliminated from Africa with vaccination and improved sanitation and access to safe drinking water. This latter measure may also reduce the incidence of viral hepatitis E [36, 37].

In order to make vaccination against HAV feasible for developing countries, it is necessary to evaluate effective and cost-effective strategies. Vizzotti et al. [38] evaluated the impact of single-dose vaccination in Argentina and found an impressive decline in hepatitis A cases accompanied by a decrease in medical and nonmedical costs in the first 5 years. The authors then suggested that this could be a simpler and less costly strategy thus becoming an economically viable alternative to other countries where hepatitis A is also endemic.

9. Future perspectives

Since both the world population and the life expectancy are increasing, it's imperative that new techniques, fast, accessible, and sensitive ones, are developed in order to guarantee accurate diagnosis and proper treatment to anyone who is suffering from a disease. With new technologies being released in a daily basis and several researches being done in fields like molecular diagnostics, immunodiagnostics, and gene therapy, it's possible that this goal may be achieved within the following decades.

So as to improve the diagnosis of hepatitis and several other diseases, either through the detection of pathogens or elements present due to the host's immune response, it's essential that new, highly sensitive tests become available in healthcare facilities, especially in endemic regions.

One possibility is to use new techniques that are being developed and allow the detection of antibodies. One example is the capacitive immunosensor developed to detect anti-Zika virus and anti-chikungunya virus antibodies in low concentrations using microwire electrodes [39].

Another possibility is to use the CRISPR-Cas technology to detect the pathogen's genetic material. This technique was developed based on the analysis of a specific defense mechanism of bacteria and archaea, organisms in which clusters of regularly interspaced short palindromic repeats (CRISPR), a specific region of the DNA, are transcribed into CRISPR RNA (crRNA) when they are infected by viruses [40, 41]. When the crRNA and the trans-activating crRNA (tracrRNA) associate with Cas9, an enzyme, the crRNA-Cas9 complex will then target a foreign DNA and cut it [40, 41].

Studies have shown that, through modification, the CRISPR-Cas complex is capable of targeting RNA [42] and adapting to different intracellular environments, such as the eukaryotic one [43]. Other experiments with CRISPR-Cas demonstrate that it can detect both Zika virus and dengue virus, RNA viruses [44]. Besides, this last analysis has also shown that a test based on this technique would be fast and sensitive and the costs would be low [44].

Regarding the treatment, some studies have shown that genome editing using the CRISPR-Cas system might also allow the development of effective antiviral therapies. Experiments done in vitro using human cells demonstrate that this system can target herpesvirus and provide either clearance of some strains of this virus or cause decay in other strains' replication [45]. Another work, by demonstrating that the CRISPR-Cas system was able to inhibit the accumulation of hepatitis B virus (HBV) DNA in human cells, has shown that this system has the capacity to be developed into an effective therapy for viral diseases [46].

Nevertheless, to ensure a decrease in the number of people infected with hepatitis, it's also important to develop strategies to prevent the spread of the virus. Since hepatitis A is transmitted through a fecal-oral pathway, to achieve this goal, it's essential that the water used by the population receives proper treatment in order to guarantee that all the pathogenic organisms are eliminated. In this context, water and sanitation projects developed by humanitarian organizations can contribute to the decrease in the number of people infected with fecal-oral transmitted diseases.

Some examples are the water safety plans (WSPs), created by the World Health Organization, and the Sustainable Development Goal 6, created by the United Nations. The former focusses on assembling a team that will develop a WSP considering all the hazardous events that can affect the safety of a water supply so as to determine and validate control measures that will be used to develop and implement improvements, which ensure that the drinking water supply is safe and accepted by the population [47]. The latter sets the goals for the following decades and analyzes indicators in order to monitor and promote the implementation of plans of action made to ensure universal and equitable access to safe and affordable drinking water for all, access to adequate and equitable sanitation, hygiene for all, end open defecation [48], and several other measures that can help control fecal-oral transmitted diseases.

10. Conclusion

Hepatitis A is a viral disease whose prevention is possible through improvements in basic sanitation and vaccination of the population. The vaccine provides good protection and is recommended in two doses for children, starting at the age of 1 year. The efficacy of the single-dose vaccine has been reported between people traveling to exotic locations and then by developing countries that have adopted this single-dose schedule. In those places where the single-dose schedule has been adopted, a surveillance system should be in place to determine whether the booster dose will be necessary over the long term. Patients with hepatitis A present evolution to the healing in the majority of the cases, but it is necessary to be aware that, in rare occasions, they can develop acute hepatic insufficiency, which is associated to greater morbimortality.

Conflict of interest

The authors declare no conflict of interest.

Author details

Julia Teixeira Rodrigues, Priscila Menezes Ferri Liu and Adriana Teixeira Rodrigues*
Federal University of Minas Gerais (UFMG), Belo Horizonte, Brazil

*Address all correspondence to: adrianatr92@gmail.com

References

[1] Matheny SC, Kingery JE. University of Kentucky College of Medicine, Lexington, Kentucky. American Family Physician. 2012;**86**(11):1027-1034

[2] Brundage SC, Fitzpatrick AN. Hepatitis A. American Family Physician. 2006;**73**(12):2162-2168

[3] Cristina J, Costa-Matiioli M. Genetic variability and molecular evolution of Hepatitis A virus. Virus Research. 2007;**127**(2):151-157. DOI: 10.1016/j.virusres.2007.01.005

[4] Acheson D, Fiore AE. Hepatitis A transmitted by food. Clinical Infectious Diseases. 2004;**38**(5):705-715. DOI: 10.1086/381671

[5] Kramer A, Schwebke I, Kampf G. How long do nosocomial pathogens persist on inanimate surfaces? A systematic review. BMC Infectious Diseases. 2006;**6**:130

[6] Ferreira CT, Silveira TR. Hepatites virais: Aspectos da epidemiologia e da prevenção. Revista Brasileira de Epidemiologia. 2004;**7**(4):473-487. DOI: 10.1590/S1415-790X2004000400010

[7] Mutsch M et al. Hepatitis A virus infections in travelers, 1988-2004. Clinical Infectious Diseases. 2006;**42**(4):490-497

[8] WHO (World Health Organization). Hepatitis A. 2018. Available from: https://www.who.int/news-room/fact-sheets/detail/hepatitis-a [Accessed: 20 June 2019]

[9] Lemon SM et al. Type A viral hepatitis: A summary and update on the molecular virology, epidemiology, pathogenesis and prevention. Journal of Hepatology. 2018;**68**:167-184

[10] Efrain E et al. Cellular entry and uncoating of naked and quasi-enveloped human hepatoviruses. eLife. 2019;**8**:e43983. DOI: 10.7554/eLife.43983

[11] Tanton BN, editor. Hepatitis viruses: Virology and epidemiology. In: Tropical Gastroenterology. New Delhi: New Elsevier; 2008. 261 p

[12] Cuthbert JA. Hepatitis A: Old and new. Clinical Microbiology Reviews. 2001;**14**(1):38-58

[13] Murray PR, Rosenthal KS, Pfaller MA, editors. Virus da hepatite. In: Microbiologia Médica. 7th ed. Vol. 2014. Rio de Janeiro: Elsevier. 1115-1121 p

[14] Maier K et al. Human gamma interferon production by cytotoxic T lymphocytes sensitized during hepatitis A virus infection. Journal of Virology. 1988;**62**:3756-3763

[15] Zhou Y et al. Dominance of the $CD4^{+}$ T helper cell response during acute resolving hepatitis A virus infection. Journal of Experimental Medicine. 2012;**209**(8):1481-1492

[16] Baba M et al. Cytolytic activity of natural killer cells and lymphokine activated killer cells against hepatitis A virus infected fibroblasts. Journal of Clinical & Laboratory Immunology. 1993;**40**(2):47-60

[17] Pereira FEL, Gonçalves CS. Hepatite A. Revista da Sociedade Brasileira de Medicina Tropical. 2003;**36**(3):387-400

[18] Dagan R et al. Incidence of hepatitis A in Israel following universal immunization of toddlers. Journal of the American Medical Association. 2005;**294**(2):202-210. DOI: 10.1001/jama.294.2.202

[19] Luxemburger C, Dutta AK. Overlapping epidemiologies of hepatitis

A and typhoid fever: The needs of the traveler. Journal of Travel Medicine. 2005;**12**(1):S12

[20] Secretaria de Vigilância em Saúde e Ministério da Saúde. Boletim Epidemiológico. 2018;**49**(31). Available from: http://portalarquivos2.saude.gov.br/images/pdf/2018/julho/05/Boletim-Hepatites-2018.pdf [Accessed: 23 June 2019]

[21] Doshani M et al. Recommendations of the advisory committee on immunization practices for use of hepatitis A vaccine for persons experiencing homelessness. MMWR. Morbidity and Mortality Weekly Report. 2019;**68**:153-156

[22] Pereira FEL, Gonçalves CS. Hepatitis A. Revistada Sociedade Brasileirade Medicina Tropical. 2003;**36**(3):387-400

[23] CDC (Center of Disease Control). Hepatitis A, Acute. Case Definition. 2019. Available from https://wwwn.cdc.gov/nndss/conditions/hepatitis-a-acute/case-definition/2019/ [Accessed: 30 May 2019]

[24] Jayakumar S et al. Fulminant viral hepatitis. Critical Care Clinics. 2013;**29**:677-697. DOI: 10.1016/j.ccc.2013.03.013

[25] DynaMed [Internet]. Ipswich (MA): EBSCO Information Services. 1995. Record No. 900055, Acute liver failure; [updated 2018 Nov 30]. Available from: http://www.dynamed.com/login.aspx?direct=true&site=DynaMed&id=900055 Registration and login required [Accessed: 20 June 2019]

[26] Leikin JB. Current and prospective therapies for acute liver failure. Disease-a-Month. 2018;**64**(12):492. DOI: 10.1016/j.disamonth.2018.10.001

[27] Barbosa PSH et al. Nutrition assessment and support of children with cholestasis. Revista Médica de Minas Gerais. 2013;**23**(Supl 2):S34-S40. DOI: 10.5935/2238-3182.2013S006

[28] Departamento de Doenças de Condições Crônicas e Infecções Sexualmente Transmissíveis do Ministério da Saúde do Brasil. Available from: http://www.aids.gov.br/pt-br/publico-geral/o-que-sao-hepatites/hepatite [Accessed: 24 July 2019]

[29] Mayorga PO et al. Efficacy of virosome hepatitis A vaccine in young children in Nicaragua: Randomized placebo-controlled trial. The Journal of Infectious Diseases. 2003;**188**:671-677

[30] Nelson NP, Link-Gelles R, Hofmeister MG, et al. Update: Recommendations of the advisory committee on immunization practices for use of hepatitis A vaccine for postexposure prophylaxis and for preexposure prophylaxis for international travel. MMWR. Morbidity and Mortality Weekly Report. 2018;**67**:1216-1220

[31] Iwarson S et al. Excellent booster response 4 to 8 years after a single primary dose of an inactivated hepatitis A vaccine. Journal of Travel Medicine. 2004;**11**:120-121

[32] Hatz C et al. Successful memory response following a booster dose with a virosome-formulated hepatitis a vaccine delayed up to 11 years. Clinical and Vaccine Immunology. 2011;**18**:885-887

[33] Vacchino MN. Incidence of hepatitis A in Argentina after vaccination. Journal of Viral Hepatitis. 2008;**15**(2):47-50

[34] Contents 261 WHO position paper on hepatitis A vaccines—June 2012. Weekly Epidemiological Record. 2012;**87**:261-276. Available from: http://www.who.int/wer [Accessed: 13 June 2019]

[35] Ministério da Saúde e Secretaria de Vigilância em Saúde Departamento de Vigilância Epidemiológica Coordenação Geral do Programa Nacional de Imunizações. Informe Técnico da Introdução da Vacina Adsorvida Hepatite A (inativada). Brasilia. 2014. Available from: http://portalarquivos2.saude.gov.br/images/pdf/2015/junho/26/Informe-t--cnico-vacina-hepatite-A-junho-2014.pdf [Accessed: 18 June 2019]

[36] ONU News. Meta da África é eliminar a hepatite viral até 2030. Available from: https://news.un.org/pt/story/2016/08/1560571-meta-da-africa-e-eliminar-hepatite-viral-ate-2030 [Accessed: 30 June 2019]

[37] WHO. Mensagem da Directora Regional da OMS para a África, Dr.ª Matshidiso Moeti, por ocasião do Dia Mundial contra a Hepatite. 2017. Available from: https://afro.who.int/pt/regional-director/speeches-messages/mensagem-da-directora-regional-da-oms-para-africa-dra-0 [Accessed: 30 June 2019]

[38] Vizzotti C et al. Economic analysis of the single-dose immunization strategy against hepatitis A in Argentina. Vaccine. 2015;**33S**:A227-A232. DOI: 10.1016/j.vaccine.2014.12.077

[39] Wang L et al. An ultra-sensitive capacitive microwire sensor for pathogen-specific serum antibody responses. Biosensors and Bioelectronics. 2019;**131**:46-52

[40] Doudna JA, Charpentier E. The new frontier of genome engineering with CRISPR-Cas9. Science. 2014;**346**(6213): 12580961-12580969. DOI: 10.1126/science.1258096. Available from https://innovativegenomics.org/wp-content/uploads/2016/06/Doudna-Charpentier-Science-2014.pdf [Accessed: 23 July 2019]

[41] Barrangou R, Doudna JA. Applications of CRISPR technologies in research and beyond. Nature Biotechnology. 2016;**34**:933-941

[42] O'Connell MR et al. Programmable RNA recognition and cleavage by CRISPR/Cas9. Nature. 2014;**516**(7530):263-266

[43] Price AA et al. Cas9-mediated targeting of viral RNA in eukaryotic cells. Proceedings of the National Academy of Sciences of the United States of America. 2015;**112**(19):6164-6169

[44] Gootenberg JS et al. Nucleic acid detection with CRISPR-Cas13a/C2c2. Science. 2017;**356**(6336):438-442

[45] van Diemen FR, Kruse EM, Hooykaas MJG, Bruggeling CE, Schürch AC, van Ham PM, et al. CRISPR/Cas9-mediated genome editing of herpesviruses limits productive and latent infections. PLoS Pathogens. 2016;**12**(6):e1005701. DOI: 10.1371/journal.ppat.1005701

[46] Kennedy EM et al. Suppression of hepatitis B virus DNA accumulation in chronically infected cells using a bacterial CRISPR/Cas RNA-guided DNA endonuclease. Virology. 2015;**476**:196-205

[47] Bartram J et al. Water Safety Plan Manual: Step by Step Risk Management for Drinking-water Supplies. Geneva: World Health Organization; 2009. Available from: https://apps.who.int/iris/handle/10665/75141 [Accessed: 23 July 2019]

[48] United Nations. Economic and Social Council. Agenda items 5(a) and 6, May 2019. Available from: https://sustainabledevelopment.un.org/hlpf/2019/ [Accessed: 23 July 2019]

Chapter 6

Antiviral Natural Products against Hepatitis-A Virus

Damian Chukwu Odimegwu
and Uzochukwu Gospel Ukachukwu

Abstract

The review on antiviral anti-hepatitis A virus agents is warranted given the importance of hepatitis A virus (HAV) as a human pathogen. Novel antiviral drugs have been sourced from natural agents and developed into products for management of viral infections. The role of purified natural products in treatment and as adjunctives in the management of HAV infections is clearly plausible. Treatments against Hepatitis A virus infection is currently limited. In this chapter, the antiviral natural products against hepatitis-A virus (HAV), their sources as well as their treatment approach and their application have been discussed. The antiviral natural products could be sourced generally from plants, herbs and animals. These natural agents have been shown to demonstrate substantial antiviral activity against HAV and could target various stages of the viral life cycle, replication, assemblage, release, as well as targeting virus-host specific interactions.

Keywords: hepatitis A, antiviral, natural products, infections

1. Introduction

The role of purified natural products in prophylaxis, palliative and curative treatment of myriad diseases of bacterial, fungal and viral origin cannot be overemphasized. Novel antiviral drugs have been sourced from natural agents and developed into products for prophylactic and therapeutic purposes [1]. These natural agents have been shown to demonstrate antiviral activity by interfering with viral life cycle, replication, assemblage, release, as well as targeting virus-host specific interactions [1]. Antiviral natural products can be sourced generally from plants or herbs, microbes, animals and humans. In this chapter, the antiviral natural products against hepatitis-A virus (HAV), their sources as well as their treatment approach and their application were adequately discussed.

2. Therapeutic anti-HAV natural products

Hepatitis A virus is among the pathogens that find their way into the human system through ingestion of food contaminated with them, and most of these food-borne viruses lack licensed antivirals. Vaccine development and immunization against several viruses including hepatitis A virus lack preventive and efficient antiviral therapies, as they are often challenged by counter-production of viral escape mutants that evade the immune system [1]. Also, the development of efficient and low-cost vaccines for economically unprivileged countries will be difficult, including countries with low prevalence where vaccine is recommended only for high-risk individuals [2]. Post-exposure of the human system to viral infections requires an efficient therapeutic approach to clear infections off the human system. It is imperative to develop effective antiviral therapeutic agents against these viruses, and interest in the employment of natural products as effective antiviral therapeutic agents has widely increased.

Flavonoids, polyphenols, saponin, proanthocyanins, polysaccharides, organic acids, proteins, polypeptides, and essential oils obtained from plant, animals or microorganisms can control and eradicate food-borne viral infections including hepatitis A [3, 4]. Over the past two decades, much effort has been aimed at identifying natural products, mostly of plant origin, to control food-borne viruses. Extracts from natural plants potentially have several applications, not limited to increasing the safety of food products and enhancing their quality, but also to serve as natural antiviral agents. For instance, these extracts possess several natural compounds that have been reported to demonstrate virucidal activity against surrogates of the human novovirus, a known food-borne virus [5]. In this section, we will discuss the antiviral therapeutic activities of several natural products and herbal medicines against hepatitis A viral infection.

2.1 Plant-based

2.1.1 Green tea extract

Green tea extract (GTE) is produced from the leaves of cultivated evergreen tea plant, *Camellia sinensis* L., of the family Theaceae [6]. It is rich in polyphenols and proanthocyanidins, and has been widely used to nutritionally enrich various food and beverages due to reports about its diverse health benefits such as possessing antioxidant, anti-inflammatory, and anti-carcinogenic properties [7–9]. Studies have revealed that GTE exhibits inhibitory properties against a wide variety of food-borne pathogens [10, 11]. Chemical composition of GTE includes mainly catechins, a group of flavonoids [12] that possess antimicrobial properties on a wide spectrum of Gram-positive and Gram-negative bacteria [11]. In a study, catechins such as epigallocatechin-3-gallate (EGCG) and epicatechin gallate (ECG), contained in GTE demonstrated the strongest antiviral properties [13], and also exhibited significant antiviral properties when encapsulated within chitosan electrosprayed microcapsules [14].

Recent *in vitro* study revealed that GTE demonstrated excellent antiviral activity against hepatitis A virus under controlled conditions of concentration, pH, temperature and also time exposure. It was shown that 5 mg/ml GTE incubated with the viral suspension for 2 h at 37°C and pH of 7.2 observed that there was complete inactivation of the virus in the suspension [6]. Findings suggested that GTE antiviral activity thrived better under increasing alkaline conditions. GTE has also been evaluated as a natural sanitizer of farm produce, demonstrating that HAV titers in lettuce and spinach were drastically reduced after 30 min treatment with 10 mg/ml GTE. Hence GTE holds promise for food-borne viral infection control through disinfection of food produce before consumption. Although the antiviral mechanisms of GTE have not yet been elucidated, some extrapolations could be drawn from the action of EGCG on viruses as it is the chief constituent compound in GTE [14, 15]. EGCG has high affinity for viral surface proteins but binds nonspecifically to them.

Therefore it exhibits its antiviral activity against a wide variety of enveloped and non-enveloped viruses by interfering with viral attachment to cell membrane receptors upon binding to them; thus, HAV infection could be curbed by GTE via similar mechanism.

2.1.2 Grape seed extract

Grape seed extract (GSE), *Vitis vinifera*, is generally obtained as a by-product of the grape juice and wine industry during processing of grapes [16]. It is reported to possess diverse bioactive principles including anthocyanins, flavonoids, proanthocyanidins, polyphenols, procyanidins and resveratrol, a derivative of stilbene [17]. The antioxidative, anti-inflammatory, cardioprotective, hepatoprotective, neuroprotective, and antimicrobial properties of these compounds make the extract to exhibit impressive pharmacological and therapeutic benefits [18].

GSE demonstrates antimicrobial activity against many food-borne bacterial pathogens including *Listeria monocytogenes*, *Staphylococcus aureus*, methicillin-resistant *S. aureus* (MRSA), *Escherichia coli* O157:H7, *Salmonella enterica* serovar Enteritidis, and *S. typhimurium* [19–21]. Moreover, studies have reported the antiviral activities of GSE against some food-borne viruses including hepatitis A virus (HAV), human norovirus surrogates (feline calicivirus (FCV-F9)) and murine norovirus (MNV-1) [22, 23]. Under simulated gastrointestinal conditions, GSE reduced the HAV titer to undetectable levels in a dose-dependent fashion at varied temperatures (room temperature, 37°C) and time not exceeding 24 h. Emphatically, 2 mg/ml GSE drastically reduced HAV titer among other food-borne viruses to undetectable levels in intestinal fluid after 6 h.

However, this success may not be reproducible in the human system as the HAV strain, HM175, used during the study was a lab-adapted strain that was not sensitive to low pH as observed in the wild type strain. Again, some studies showed that GSE anti-HAV activity decreased in the presence of increasing concentrations of 0.02 and 0.2% dried milk or lettuce extract, where a higher dose is required to inactivate viral replication [24]. This implies that proteins could interfere with GSE antiviral activity and consequently decreases its effectiveness for treatments. Also, at concentrations ranging from 0.25 to 1 mg/ml GSE was said to diminish food-borne viral contamination levels on food produce (lettuce and peppers) without causing notable color changes on them. Therefore, GSE could be considered as a control measure for hepatitis A virus contamination on food produce before consumption, though may require a synergistic approach to combat persistent contamination of food produce.

The antiviral mechanisms of GSE are not yet well expounded. However, some studies suggest that resveratrol (RV), a nonflavonoid polyphenol found in grapes modulate some intracellular signaling pathways of the influenza virus [25]. In a study evaluating the effect of GSE on the adsorption and replicativity of HAV, it was revealed that treatment of the host cells with GSE prior to viral infection caused significant decline in HAV titer [26]. Post-viral infection of the host cells showed that HAV titers decreased insignificantly. This implies that GSE may have a moderate antiviral effect on adsorption of HAV on the host cells but with less effect on its replication [26]. Likewise, GSE was reported to down-regulate the expression of HIV entry coreceptors, implying that GSE may interrupt the binding of the virus to the cell receptors and in turn prevent HIV entry into normal lymphocytes [27]. Presently, GSE appears not to cause any structural damage to the viral capsid of HAV, rather it is more likely to exert greater antiviral activity by potentially blocking the host cell receptors and consequently prevents viral entry, replication, and infection.

2.1.3 Egyptian red sea seagrass extract

Seagrass is a critical part of the marine ecosystem and is generally distributed along the tropical and temperate coastal zones of the world [28]. It was said to be the only marine flowering plant that completes its lifecycle in sea water and often lives entirely submerged [29]. It is of ecological importance and is employed in folklore medicine for therapeutic purposes [30, 31]. The Egyptian Red Sea seagrass, *Thalassodendron ciliatum*, is said to be one of the longest and most common sea grasses along the Egyptian Red Sea. Its leaves are characterized by many 'tannin cells' more than in any other sea grass [32], which infers that it possesses a high phenolic content.

Compounds isolated from the sea grass crude extract have been shown to exhibit antioxidant and cytotoxic activities [28]. The crude extract demonstrated 100% inhibition of hepatitis A (HAV) and Herpes Simplex (HSV-1) viruses at 20 μg/mL. The antiviral activity of the crude extract against HAV was lost by fractionation, which could be explained by the synergistic action of several compounds in the crude extract [28]. Moreover, knowledge about the mechanism of anti-HAV activity of *T. ciliatum* has not yet been elucidated. Further studies are required to evaluate the toxicity of *T. ciliatum* on humans after consumption as food supplement or on formulation as a therapeutic drug against HAV.

2.1.4 Essential oils

Essential oils (EOs) are aromatic oily liquids derived from plant materials such as flowers, buds, seeds, leaves, branches, bark, grass, wood, fruit, and roots. Production of essential oils is majorly by steam distillation or by other methods such as solvent-heat extraction, pressing, fermentation or enfleurage [33]. Chemical components contained in these essential oils have been shown to be effective in combating pathogens [34, 35]. Few essential oils have been tested for their antiviral activities against food-borne viruses, particularly for HAV [36].

The anti-HAV activity of essential oils obtained from lemon (*Citrus limon*), sweet orange (*Citrus sinensis*), grapefruit (*Citrus paradisi*), and rosemary cineole (*Rosmarinus officinalis*) have been reported [33]. Essential oils belonging to the genus *Citrus* contain 85–99% of volatile compounds such as sesquiterpenes, monoterpene (limonene), and hydrocarbons, with their oxygenated products including aldehydes (citral), acids, ketones, alcohols (linalool), and esters [37]. *Rosmarinus officinalis* of the family, *Lamiaceae*, is generally applied during the preparation of some European cuisine and is also used as a medicinal plant, because of the strong antiseptic properties, antibacterial and antioxidant activities of it's essential oil [38]; rosemary oil is also used as a natural food preservative [39, 40].

Essential oil treatment of ATCC/HM-175 strain of HAV propagated in Frp3 cells revealed that after an hour incubation at room temperature, the greatest reduction in cell infectivity was observed for rosemary cineole EO, followed by grapefruit and lemon EOs, while orange EO, although reducing HAV infectivity was not statistically significant [33]. Orange and grapefruit EOs were found to be cytotoxic for Frp3 cells at concentrations that exceeded 0.1%, while lemon and rosemary cineole EOs were cytotoxic at concentrations exceeding 0.5% and 0.05%, respectively. Studies have also revealed that treatment of contaminated berries with all four EOs from lemon, orange, grapefruit and rosemary cineole reduced the viral titer of HAV at room temperature. Essential oil from rosemary cineole was shown to be the most effective, as it significantly reduced the HAV titer on the berries followed by essential oils from grapefruit and lemon respectively [33]. Anti-HAV activity of essential oil from orange was not significant though there was a reduction in the

HAV titer on the berries. However, application of these essential oils alone may not be sufficient to decontaminate soft fruits (berries) laden with higher viral (HAV) loads [33]. Therefore, it is imperative that the essential oils be considered for use in food sterilization in combination with other treatments. It is also necessary to evaluate the minimum time it takes for EOs to reduce the maximum HAV loads on food produce so that adequate awareness is made to individuals to achieve food product safety before consumption [33]. Moreover, the mechanisms of anti-HAV activity of EOs have not yet been elucidated.

2.1.5 Korean red ginseng extract and ginsenosides

Ginseng (*Panax ginseng* Meyer) is a famous medicinal herb that has been used for over 5000 years in Korea and China [41]. Ginseng contains myriad bioactive components including, ginsenosides, phytosterols, polysaccharides, polyacetylenes, polyacetylenic alcohols, fatty acids and peptides [42]. There exists already documentations on the anti-stress, anti-carcinogenic, anti-inflammatory, antioxidant, anti-bacterial, anti-viral and anti-fungal activities of ginseng [42–44]. Furthermore, ginseng demonstrates useful activity on endocrine diseases, cardiovascular diseases and the immune system [45]. During processing, Red ginseng is usually steamed and fermented with skinned ginseng and this alters the composition saponin contained in it when done repeatedly [46]. Red ginseng has been shown to possess anti-cancer, anti-diabetic, anti-obesity and immunomodulatory properties [3, 4]. Likewise zidovudine, red ginseng has also been applied as a therapeutic supplement for the treatment of patients with human immunodeficiency virus [47].

Studies have shown that red ginseng extract and its ginsenosides inactivate food borne viruses such as the human norovirus (huNoV) surrogates (feline calicivirus and murine norovirus) [43]. A plaque assay performed on FRhK-4 cell lines pre-treated and co-treated with varied concentrations of Korean red ginseng (KRG) extract and purified ginsenosides (Rg1 and Rb1) showed that after inoculation of HAV HM-175 strain on the cell lines, KRG and the ginsenosides reduced significantly the HAV concentration [3, 4]. Korean red ginseng's extract demonstrated cytotoxicity at concentration above 10 μg/mL, while the purified ginsenosides showed no cytotoxic activity even up to 40 μg/mL. Although co-treatment of cell lines with KRG and the ginsenosides exhibited significant reduction of HAV concentration in the study, anti-HAV activity of the pretreated cell lines was quite higher [3, 4]. Hence, pretreatment with ginseng may be effective in preventing HAV infection. Also co-treatment of cell lines with KRG and the ginsenosides may be evaluated in further study using *in vivo* models.

The anti-HAV mechanisms of KRG extract and its ginsenosides are not clearly defined. However, reports from studies have shown that HAV-infected FRhK-4 cells activate the 2′-5′ oligoadenylate synthetase/RNaseL pathway [48]. Activation of RNase L degrades viral RNA and cellular single-stranded RNA; hence, KRG extract and its ginsenosides may tour a similar path. In addition, previous studies have reported that ginseng polysaccharides and ginsenosides have the capacity to boost the production of cytokines via stimulation of immune cells [3, 4]. Interferons induced by this pathway also contribute to the antiviral response.

2.1.6 Blueberry juice and blueberry proanthocyanidins

Blueberries are said to contain about 88–261 mg of proanthocyanidin/100 g of edible portion according to the USDA database for flavonoid content (USDA Database for the proanthocyanidin Content of Selected Foods, August 2004). Again, blue berries possess some other structurally related polyphenols such as anthocyanins and flavonoids [49]. Blueberry juice and its polyphenols have been found to have promising health benefits which include their cardioprotective, neuroprotective, anticarcinogenic, antibacterial, and antiviral properties [50]. Ethanol and water extracts of blueberries were reported to decrease *Listeria monocytogenes* by 5.90 log CFU/ml at 24 ppm and 37°C after 24 h *in-vitro* [51]. Also, 0.4 g/L gallic acid from blueberries caused a reduction in of *E. coli* O157:H7 titer in addition to the disruption of its cell-membrane after 24 h at 37°C *in-vitro* [52]. In addition, in a hepatitis C virus replicon cell system, methanol extract fraction of blueberry leaves (0.112–2200 lg/ml) was shown to suppress hepatitis C virus (HCV) subgenomic expression at 37°C after 72 h [53].

Recent study evaluated the antiviral activities of Blueberry juice and its proanthocyanidins (B-type) against HAV and some of human norovirus surrogates [50]. It was shown that in suspension, HAV titers were reduced by proanthocyanidins (2 and 5 mg/ml) to undetectable levels after 30 min, and after 3 h by 1 mg/ml proanthocyanidins. HAV titer was only reduced to by 2 log PFU/ml with Blue berry juice at pH 2.8 and 37°C after 24 h [50]. FRhK4 cells pre-infected and post-infected with HAV (strain; HM175) were also investigated for viral adsorption and replication upon treatment with the Blueberry juice and isolated proanthocyanidins [50]. The Blue berry proanthocyanidins showed promising preventive capacity as it moderately reduced HAV infectivity in the pre-infected cells but did not affect the replication of HAV in the post-infected cells. Hence, the Blue berry proanthocyanidins interrupt HAV binding and entry much more than it can limit its replication in the host cells; suggesting that it's antiviral efficacy is more preventive than therapeutic.

2.1.7 Aqueous extracts of Hibiscus sabdariffa *calyces*

Hibiscus sabdariffa, belonging to the family, Malvaceae, is an annual tropical or subtropical shrub species found in countries including Mexico, Sudan, India, and Thailand [54]. It is commonly called 'roselle' and is used for ornamental purposes, and the red calyces of *H. sabdariffa* are often used in the preparation of cold or hot beverages [55]. The calyces are said to be rich in bioactive compounds like anthocyanins, saponins, phenolic acids, organic acids and alkaloids [56]. Presence of organic acids like malic and tartaric acids identified in the calyces, possess a low pH of approximately 2–2.5 [54]. Aqueous extracts of the calyces are considered generally as safe and are approved for use as food additives by the U.S. Food and Drug Administration (21 CFR 172.510) in the flavoring of beverages [22, 23]. The calyces of *H. sabdariffa* are reported to possess a wide range of health benefits including antioxidant, anticancer, cardioprotective, anti-diabetic, and antimicrobial effects [57–59]. Protocatechuic acid (PCA), an essential component of *H. sabdariffa* has been shown to be the component responsible for its antimicrobial activity [60]. Another chemical component of the genus Hibiscus, known as Ferulic acid (FA) has also been reported to exhibit antimicrobial properties and antifilarial activity against *Setaria cervi* [61, 62].

Recent study evaluated the antiviral activity of *H. sabdariffa* against human novovirus surrogates and HAV. Findings revealed that aqueous extracts of calyces of *H. sabdariffa* (100 and 40 mg/ml) reduced HAV titer in suspension to undetectable levels at 37°C after 24 h [22, 23]. However, PCA demonstrated a moderate antiviral effect on HAV as it significantly reduced the HAV titer in suspension but not to undetectable levels. Pre- and post-infection assays with the aqueous extract of the calyces of *H. sabdariffa* (5 mg/ml) demonstrated no notable change in titres observed for HAV [22, 23]. Higher concentrations (40 and 100 mg/ml) of the aqueous extract was found to be cytotoxic to the host cell lines when added; observation for visual cytopathic effect under the light microscope showed that cells were peeling off [22, 23]. It is likely the aqueous extract is effective for alleviating viral burden; however this has not yet been substantiated as more studies into model food systems and simulation of gastrointestinal tract conditions to test the efficacy of the extracts under *in vivo* conditions are required.

2.1.8 4-phenylcoumarin derivatives

Coumarin was first isolated from tonka beans, *Dipteryx odoranta*, also called Coumarou and biological activities of thousands of natural coumarins from plants, bacteria and fungi and chemical synthesis have been reported [63]. Coumarin and its derivatives have been used to manufacture drugs serving as anticoagulants including warfarin, acenocoumarin and phenprocoumon, and also for production of novobiocin, a potent inhibitor of bacterial DNA gyrase [63]. Coumarins (2H-chromen-2-ones) are recognized as a privileged bioactive scaffold for designing new agents with high affinity and specificity to various molecular targets [64], especially as antiviral agents [65]. In recent years, 4-Phenylcoumarins (neoflavones) which are bio-isosteres of flavonoids, have been of much interest as lead target structure for the discovery of new antiviral agents [66, 67].

A more recent study demonstrated that some coumarin derivatives possess anti-HAV activity. Newly modified 4-phenylcoumarin-based compounds were developed and evaluated for inhibition of 3C proteases [63]. Similar to other picornaviruses, HAV genome encodes a key processing protease, known as HAV 3C protease (HAV $3C^{pro}$), which is a nonstructural cysteine protein responsible for the cleavage process within the viral polyprotein (250 kDa) that is critical for the replication process [63]. These proteases are responsible for processing the polyprotein precursor and also cleaving specific cellular factors needed for transcription and translation processes as well as nucleo-cytoplasmic trafficking in order to alter cell physiology to enhance viral replication; thus $3C^{pro}$ is vital to viral life cycle, making the viral 3C proteases choice targets for antiviral therapy [63]. Evaluation of the target compounds for their antiviral activity against hepatitis A virus revealed that the derivative, 1-(2-(2-Oxo-4-phenyl-2H-chromen-7-yloxy)acetyl) 4-ethylthiosemicarbazide had the most potent virucidal activity (IC_{50} = 3.1 μg/ml, TI = 83). The derivatives, 2-(2-Oxo-4-phenyl-2H-chromen-7-yloxy)-N′-(1-(4-chlorophenyl) ethylidene)acetohydrazide and 2-(2-Oxo-4-phenyl-2H-chromen-7-yloxy)-N′-(1-(4-bromophenyl)ethylidene)acetohydrazide demonstrated the strongest virustatic effects against HAV adsorption and replication, respectively (IC_{50} = 8.5 μg/ml, TI =88; IC_{50} = 10.7 μg/ml, TI = 91). Furthermore, studies reported that the three newly derived compounds were tested against HAV 3C protease and they exhibited remarkable inhibition effects (Ki = 1.903, 0.104 and 0.217 μM, respectively) indicating strong binding to HAV $3C^{pro}$ [63]. Also, the three compounds were docked within the pocket site of HAV 3C protease (PDB code: 2HAL) which illustrated that they had strong H-profiles with the amino acids Gly170 and Cys172. Findings suggested that the target compounds inhibited virus infection through the interrupting virus adsorption to the cell surface. This may have occurred via blocking of the cellular surface receptors by the target compounds which consequently led to an anti-HAV effect. Deduction from the post-treatment assay suggested that the target compounds inhibited the activities of some viral enzymes needed to complete the replication cycle or that they interfered with one or more steps in the viral life cycle.

2.1.9 Protamine, taxifolin and atropine

Protamine, a cationic peptide, is generally obtained from fish milt (spermatic cells) and is applied medically as a heparin antagonist, an injectable insulin-carrier, and recently as an antibacterial ingredient in some food products [68]. Taxifolin (dihydroquercetin) is a flavononol amply found in grapes, olive oil, citrus fruits and onions [69]. It has been shown to possess strong pharmacological activities, including antioxidative, hepatoprotective, cardioprotective, anti-diabetic, anti-inflammatory, antitumor, neuroprotective effects, and had played a remarkable role in the preclusion of Alzheimer's disease [69]. Atropine is naturally occurring compound (alkaloid) majorly found in belladonna (Solanaceae) plants. It is a muscuranic receptor antagonist and is used medically to modulate muscular contractions and dilations which consequently regulate blood flow to cells and tissues [70].

A previous study investigated the inhibitory potential of protamine, atropine and taxifolin against HAV replication in PLC/PRF/5 cells, and found out that the trio exhibited some significant but not drastic effects on HAV replication [2]. Atropine demonstrated a concentration–dependent reduction in the infectivity of HAV but the antigenicity of the virus was not affected. HAV titer was reduced at the maximum concentration of 50, 59 and 50 μg/ml of protamine, taxifolin and atropine, respectively. It was suggested that further studies be done to determine the effect of these compounds on several multiplicities of HAV infection and also investigate possible synergistic effects of these compounds with other substances that have potential for clinical use against HAV infection [2]. The mechanisms of HAV titer reduction by the compounds are not yet clearly elucidated.

3. Adjunctive anti-HAV natural products

3.1 Japanese rice-koji miso extracts

Koji, also known as *Aspergillus oryzae*, is a filamentous fungus employed by the Japanese to ferment certain kinds of food like soybeans, potatoes, rice and some other grains [71]. Miso is one of the by-products of the fermentation of Japanese rice by Koji. Miso is conventional Japanese seasoning used for preparing miso soup, a staple Japanese cuisine [71]. Previous studies showed that Japanese miso extract increases the expression of a heat-shock protein known as glucose-regulated protein 78 (GRP78) and suppresses ultraviolet C mutagenesis [72]. Some researchers observed that HAV replication was retarded upon expression of GRP78 [71]; hence GRP78 has become a potential host antiviral against HAV infection [73]. Recent post-infection assay examined miso extracts obtained from Japanese rice-koji for antiviral activity against HAV, and it was shown that the miso extracts inhibited HAV replication by enhancing the expression of GRP78 in human hepatocytes (Huh7 and PXB cells) [71]. These findings suggested that Japanese miso extracts may synergistically work as antivirals against HAV infection by partially modulating GRP78 expression [71]. Miso extracts may also serve as effective dietary supplements for the control of acute hepatitis A infection.

3.2 Korean soy sauce

Conventional Korean soy sauce is generally made with germinated soybean, salt and water [74]. The soy sauce is fermented after cooking and crushing soybean, then mold it into a block form (Meju) with concurrent addition of salt (NaCl) and water before exposing it to natural conditions [3, 4]. The percentage salt content of traditional Korean soy sauce is around 16.3–20.8% NaCl [75]. Studies have shown that soy sauce possesses diverse biological activities such as angiotensin inhibitory, anti-platelet, anticarcinogenic, and anti-oxidant activities [74]. Also, there is a report about the antibacterial activity of soy sauce against *Escherichia coli* O157:H7 [76]. The antimicrobial effects of soy sauce were attributed to the presence of a combination of ingredients and properties including NaCl, ethanol, pH, organic acids, and preservatives [74].

A study that evaluated the antiviral activity of the Korean soy sauce on HAV inoculated in raw fresh crabs (*Portunus trituberculantus*) to simulate storage conditions for homemade Ganjanggejang (a salted preserved raw seafood in Korean cuisine) revealed that there was an over 90% reduction of the HAV titer in the Ganjanggejang marinated in soy sauce containing 20% NaCl for at least 3 days [74]. Hence, the soy sauce was synergistically more effective at increasing salt concentrations. The antiviral activity of soy sauce is majorly due to the salt (NaCl) concentrations and partially attributable to its other constituents, such as ethanol, organic acids, and preservatives, and the pH of 5.11–6.98 [77]. Inhibition of HAV in crabs by NaCl in soy sauce might be due to changes in water activity which may affect virus survival [77]. In addition, antiviral mechanisms associated with NaCl may include altering the molecular structure of the viral RNA and inhibiting the viral enzymes' activity [74]. However, it's not likely that Korean soy sauce will be of relevance in clinical practice rather it may be instrumental for immediate food preservation and storage before consumption (**Table 1**).

Evaluated natural products	Concentration	Result	Proposed mechanism of action	References
Green Tea Extract	5 mg/ml for 2 h at 37°C and pH of 7.2	Complete inactivation of HAV in suspension	Interfers with viral attachment to cell membrane receptors upon binding to them	[7, 15]
Grape Seed Extract	2 mg/ml for 6 h at 37°C	Reduced HAV titer to undetectable levels under simulated gastrointestinal conditions	Interrupt the binding of HAV to the cell receptors, preventing adsorption.	[23, 24, 28]
Egyptian Red Sea Seagrass Crude Extract	20 μg/mL	100% inhibition of HAV in a plaque assay	—	[28]
Essential Oils (EO) from lemon, grapefruit and rosemary cineole	0.1% (EO from grapefruit); 0.5% (EO from lemon); 0.05% (EO from rosemary cineole)	Significant reduction in cell infectivity in the order; rosemary cineole > grapefruit > lemon.	—	[33]
Korean Red Ginseng Extract and Ginsenosides	5–10 μg/mL For 24 h at 37°C	Significant reduction of HAV titer with dose-dependent manner in pretreated FRhk-4 cells	(1) Activation of the 2′-5′oligoadenylate synthetase/RNaseL pathway; (2) boost the production of cytokines	[3–5, 49]
Blueberry Juice	pH 2.8 at 37°C for 24 h	Reduced HAV titer by 2 log PFU/ml	Interfers with HAV binding to host cells	[50]
Blueberry Proanthocyanidins	2 and 5 mg/ml for 30 min at 37°C	Reduced HAV titer to undetectable levels in suspension	Interrupt HAV binding and entry into host cells	[50]

Evaluated natural products	Concentration	Result	Proposed mechanism of action	References
Aqueous extracts of *Hibiscus sabdariffa* Calyces	100 mg/ml and 40 mg/ml at 37°C for 24 h	Reduced HAV titer to undetectable levels in suspension	—	[22, 23]
4-phenylcoumarin derivatives	10 μl at 37°C	Inhibited the activity of HAV 3C protease	Interrupt HAV adsorption on cell surface	[63]
Protamine	50 μg/ml	Reduced HAV infectivity	—	[2]
Taxifolin	59 μg/ml	Reduced HAV infectivity	—	[2]
Atropine	50 μg/ml	Reduced HAV infectivity	—	[2]
Japanese rice-koji miso extracts	—	Inhibited HAV replication	Inhibited HAV replication by enhancing the expression of GRP78 in human hepatocytes	[71]
Korean Soy Sauce	Containing 20% NaCl	over 90% reduction of the HAV titer	Inhibition of viral enzymes' activity	[74]

Table 1.
Summary of anti-HAV natural products.

4. Miscellaneous products

Duck hepatitis A virus type-1(DHAV-1) is a variant of hepatitis A virus that attacks ducks. It has been proposed that duck hepatitis A is a small animal model for the human hepatitis A [78]. It may be correct to say that antiviral agents against DHAV-1 will also demonstrate appropriate antiviral activity against human hepatitis A virus. Several natural agents have been under study to explore their antiviral potentials against DHAV-1 and they include phosphorylated *Codonopsis pilosula* polysaccharide (pCPP), Raw Rehmannia Radix Polysaccharide (RRRP), Baicalin phospholipid complex (BAPC), flavonoid combinations—baicalin-linarin-icariin-notoginsenosideR1 (BLIN).

It was reported that **RRRP** could significantly reduce mortality rate, liver lesion scoring, alleviate visual liver lesion, and decrease the alterations of plasma biochemical evaluation indexes of hepatic injury induced by DHAV-1 infection [79]. **pCPP** was also reported to demonstrate a strong inhibitory effect on DHAV-1 replication, which led to a significant decrease on the number of viral particles [80]. Studies with DHAV-1-infected ducklings treated with **BAPC** showed that it significantly inhibited DHAV-1 adsorption, replication and release [81]. Furthermore, it was reported that BAPC played anti-oxidative and immuno-supportive roles during the treatment, and that the immuno-supportive role was critical to the treatment. Another study evaluated the anti-DHAV-1 activity of a flavonoid mix, **BLIN** [82]. At 20 μg/mL, DHAV-1 inhibitory rate of BLIN at 20 μg/mL was reported to be 69.3% in duck embryonic hepatocytes. It was demonstrated that the survival rate of ducklings treated by BLIN was about 35.5%, which was remarkably higher than that of virus control (0.0%) [82]. In addition, after the treatment with BLIN, both the hepatic injury and the oxidative stress of the infected ducklings assuaged [82]. Concurrently, a significant positive correlation was said to exist between the hepatic injury indices and the oxidative stress indices.

5. Future outlook

Currently, studies exploring potential anti-HAV natural products are still emerging and had attracted little attention, possibly because a vaccine has been developed to mitigate the spread of the viral infection to a considerable length of years. However, there is need for development of more efficient and effective anti-HAV therapeutic, prophylactic and adjunctive agents, and as at now, none has been licensed. Investigations into natural products with anti-HAV hold a promising outlook as several of them have demonstrated remarkable potential to control HAV infection and replication. In addition, studies should be aimed at mimicking more closely the features of the human hepatitis A virus *in vivo* than *in vitro* so as to clearly establish the basis for the application of these natural agents in a clinical setting. There is need to develop suitable animal models that could present very similar clinical manifestations as found in humans during hepatitis A virus infection, for more accurate interpretation and correlation of outcomes from pre-clinical studies involving natural products therapy. Hopefully, studies on antiviral natural products against HAV will gain ample attention in the nearest future.

Author details

Damian Chukwu Odimegwu[1]* and Uzochukwu Gospel Ukachukwu[2]

1 Faculty of Pharmaceutical Sciences, Department of Pharmaceutical Microbiology and Biotechnology, University of Nigeria, Nsukka, Enugu State, Nigeria

2 Faculty of Biological Sciences, Department of Biochemistry, University of Nigeria, Nsukka, Enugu State, Nigeria

*Address all correspondence to: damian.odimegwu@unn.edu.ng

References

[1] Lin L, Hsu W, Lin C. Antiviral natural products and herbal medicines. Journal of Traditional and Complementary Medicine. 2014;**4**(1):24-35

[2] Biziagos E, Crance J-M, Passagot J, Deloince R. Effect of antiviral substances on hepatitis A virus replication in vitro. Journal of Medical Virology. 1987;**22**:57-66

[3] Lee DY, Chung SJ, Kim KW. Sensory characteristics of different types of commercial soy sauce. Journal of the Korean Society of Food Culture. 2013;**28**:640-650

[4] Lee MH, Lee B-H, Lee S, Choi C. Reduction of hepatitis a virus on frhk-4 cells treated with Korean red ginseng extract and ginsenosides. Journal of Food Science. 2013;**00**:M1-M4

[5] Li D, Baert L, Uyttendaele M. Inactivation of food-borne viruses using natural biochemical substances. Food Microbiology. 2013;**35**:1-9

[6] Randazzo W, Falcó-Ferrando I, Aznar R, Sánchez G. Effect of green tea extract on enteric viruses and its application as natural sanitizer. Food Microbiology. 2017;**66**:150-156. DOI: 10.1016/j.fm.2017.04.018

[7] Cooper R, Morré DJ, Morré DM. Medicinal benefits of green tea: Part I. Review of non-cancer health benefits. Journal of Alternative and Complementary Medicine. 2005;**11**:521-528

[8] Cooper R, Morré DJ, Morré DM. Medicinal benefits of green tea: Part II. Review of anticancer properties. Journal of Alternative and Complementary Medicine. 2005;**11**:639-652

[9] Xia E-Q, Deng G-F, Guo Y-J, Li H-B. Biological activities of polyphenols from grapes. International Journal of Molecular Sciences. 2010;**11**:622-646

[10] An B-J, Kwak J-H, Son J-H, Park J-M, Lee J-Y, Jo C, et al. Biological and anti-microbial activity of irradiated green tea polyphenols. Food Chemistry. 2004;**88**:549-555

[11] Gadang V, Hettiarachchy N, Johnson M, Owens C. Evaluation of antibacterial activity of whey protein isolate coating incorporated with nisin, grape seed extract, malic acid, and EDTA on a turkey frankfurter system. Journal of Food Science. 2008;**73**:M389-M394

[12] Yilmaz Y. Novel uses of catechins in foods. Trends in Food Science & Technology. 2006;**17**:64-71

[13] Dhiman RK. The green tea polyphenol, epigallocatechin-3-gallate (EGCG)—One step forward in antiviral therapy against hepatitis C virus. Journal of Clinical and Experimental Hepatology. 2011;**1**:159-160

[14] Gómez-Mascaraque LG, Sanchez G, López-Rubio A. Impact of molecular weight on the formation of electrosprayed chitosan microcapsules as delivery vehicles for bioactive compounds. Carbohydrate Polymers. 2016;**150**:121-130

[15] Steinmann J, Buer J, Pietschmann T, Steinmann E. Anti-infective properties of epigallocatechin-3-gallate (EGCG), a component of green tea. British Journal of Pharmacology. 2013;**168**:1059-1073

[16] D'Souza DH. Phytocompounds for the control of human enteric viruses. Current Opinion in Virology. 2014;**4**:44-49

[17] Jayaprakasha GK, Selvi T, Sakariah KK. Antibacterial and antioxidant activities of grape

(*Vitis vinifera*) seed extracts. Food Research International. 2003;**36**:117-122

[18] Nassiri-Asl M, Hosseinzadeh H. Review of the pharmacological effects of *Vitis vinifera* (grape) and its bioactive compounds. Phytotherapy Research. 2009;**23**:1197-1204

[19] Al-Habib A, Al-Saleh E, Safer AM, Afzal M. Bactericidal effect of grape seed extract on methicillin-resistant *Staphylococcus aureus* (MRSA). The Journal Toxicological Sciences. 2010;**35**:357-364

[20] Kao TT, Tu HC, Chang WN, Chen BH, Shi YY, Chang TC, et al. Grape seed extract inhibits the growth and pathogenicity of *Staphylococcus aureus* by interfering with dihydrofolate reductase activity and folate-mediated one-carbon metabolism. International Journal of Food Microbiology. 2010;**141**:17-27

[21] Perumalla AVS, Hettiarachchy NS. Green tea and grape seed extracts—Potential applications in food safety and quality. Food Research International. 2011;**44**:827-839

[22] Joshi SS, Dice L, D'Souza DH. Aqueous extracts of *Hibiscus sabdariffa* calyces decrease hepatitis A virus and human norovirus surrogate titers. Food and Environmental Virology. 2015;7(4):366-373

[23] Joshi SS, Su X, D'Souza DH. Antiviral effects of grape seed extract against feline calicivirus, murine norovirus, and hepatitis A virus in model food systems and under gastric conditions. Food Microbiology. 2015;**52**:1-10

[24] Li D, Baert L, Zhang D, Xia M, Zhong W, Van Coillie E, et al. Effect of grape seed extract on human norovirus GII.4 and murine norovirus 1 in viral suspensions, on stainless steel discs, and in lettuce wash water. Applied and Environmental Microbiology. 2012;**78**:7572-7578

[25] Palamara AT, Nencioni L, Aquilano K, De Chiara G, Hernandez L, Cozzolino F, et al. Inhibition of influenza A virus replication by resveratrol. The Journal of Infectious Diseases. 2005;**191**:1719-1729

[26] Su X, D'Souza DH. Grape seed extract for the control of human enteric viruses. Applied and Environmental Microbiology. 2011;**77**:3982-3987

[27] Nair MP, Kandaswami C, Mahajan S, Nair HN, Chawda R, Shanahan T, et al. Grape seed extract proanthocyanidins down regulate HIV1 entry co-receptors, CCR2b, CCR3 and CCR5 gene expression by normal peripheral blood mononuclear cells. Biological Research. 2002;**35**:421-431

[28] Hamdy A-HA, Mettwally WSA, El Fotouh MA, Rodriguez B, El-Dewany AI, El-Toumy SAA, et al. Bioactive phenolic compounds from the Egyptian Red Sea seagrass *Thalassodendron ciliatum*. Zeitschrift für Naturforschung. 2012;**67c**:291-296

[29] Short F, Carruthers T, Dennison W, Waycott M. Global seagrass distribution and diversity: A bioregional model. Journal of Experimental Marine Biology and Ecology. 2007;**350**:3-20

[30] Hemminga MA, Duarte CM. Seagrass Ecology. Cambridge: Cambridge University Press; 2000. p. 298

[31] Torre-Castro M, Rönnbäck P. Links between humans and sea grasses, an example from tropical East Africa. Ocean and Coastal Management. 2004;**47**:361-387

[32] Lipkin Y. *Thalassodendretum ciliati* in Sinai (northern Red Sea) with special reference to quantitative aspects. Aquatic Botany. 1988;**31**:125-139

[33] Battistini R, Rossini I, Ercolini C, Goria M, Callipo MR, Maurella C, et al. Antiviral activity of essential oils against hepatitis a virus in soft fruits. Food and Environmental Virology. 2019;**11**(1):90-95

[34] Ozogul Y, Kuley E, Ucar Y, Ozogul F. Antimicrobial impacts of essential oils on food borne-pathogens. Recent Patents on Food, Nutrition & Agriculture. 2015;**7**(1):53-61

[35] Piątkowska E, Rusiecka-Ziółkowska J. Influence of essential oils on infectious agents. Advances in Clinical and Experimental Medicine. 2016;**25**(5):989-995

[36] Sánchez C, Aznar R, Sánchez G. The effect of carvacrol on enteric viruses. International Journal of Food Microbiology. 2015;**192**:72-76

[37] Fisher K, Phillips C. Potential antimicrobial uses of essential oils in food: Is citrus the answer? Trends in Food Science & Technology. 2008;**19**(3):156-164

[38] Nieto G. Biological activities of three essential oils of the Lamiaceae family. Medicines (Basel). 2017;**4**(3):63

[39] Satyal P, Jones TH, Lopez EM, McFeeters RL, Ali NA, Mansi I, et al. Chemotypic characterization and biological activity of *Rosmarinus officinalis*. Food. 2017;**6**(3):20

[40] Sirocchi V, Devlieghere F, Peelman N, Sagratini G, Maggi F, Vittori S, et al. Effect of *Rosmarinus officinalis* L. essential oil combined with different packaging conditions to extend the shelf life of refrigerated beef meat. Food Chemistry. 2017;**221**: 1069-1076

[41] Yun TK. Brief introduction of *Panax ginseng* C.A. Meyer. Journal of Korean Medical Science. 2001;**16**:S3-S5

[42] Gillis CN. *Panax ginseng* pharmacology: A nitric oxide link? Biochemical Pharmacology. 1997;**54**(1):1-8

[43] Lee MH, Lee BH, Jung JY, Cheon DS, Kim KT, Choi C. Antiviral effect of Korean red ginseng extract and ginsenosides on murine norovirus and feline calicivirus as surrogates for human norovirus. Journal of Ginseng Research. 2011;**35**(4):429-435

[44] Ng TB, Wang H. Panaxagin, a new protein from Chinese ginseng possesses anti-fungal, anti-viral, translation-inhibiting and ribonuclease activities. Life Sciences. 2001;**68**(7):739-749

[45] Attele AS, Wu JA, Yuan CS. Ginseng pharmacology: Multiple constituents and multiple actions. Biochemical Pharmacology. 1999;**58**(11):1685-1693

[46] Li H, Lee JH, Ha JM. Effective purification of ginsenosides from cultured wild ginsengroots, red ginseng, and white ginseng with macroporous resins. Journal of Microbiology and Biotechnology. 2008;**18**(11):1789-1791

[47] Cho YK, Sung H, Lee HJ, Joo CH, Cho GJ. Long-term intake of Korean red ginseng in HIV-1-infected patients: Development of resistance mutation to zidovudine is delayed. International Immunopharmacology. 2001;**1**(7):1295-1305

[48] Kulka M, Calvo MS, Ngo DT, Wales SQ, Goswami BB. Activation of the 2-5OAS/RNaseL pathway in CVB1 or HAV/18f infected FRhK-4 cells does not require induction of OAS1or OAS2 expression. Virology. 2009;**388**(1):169-184

[49] Huang WY, Zhang HC, Liu WX, Li CY. Survey of antioxidant capacity and phenolic composition of blueberry, blackberry, and strawberry in Nanjing. Journal of Zhejiang University. Science. B. 2012;**13**:94-102

[50] Joshi SS, Howell AB, D'Souza DH. Reduction of enteric viruses by blueberry juice and blueberry proanthocyanidins. Food and Environmental Virology. 2016;**8**(4):235-243

[51] Park YJ, Biswas R, Phillips RD, Chen J. Antibacterial activities of blueberry and muscadine phenolic extracts. Journal of Food Science. 2011;**76**:M101-M105

[52] Lacombe A, Tadepalli S, Hwang CA, Wu VC. Phytochemicals in low bush wild blueberry inactivate *Escherichia coli* O157:H7 by damaging its cell membrane. Foodborne Pathogens and Disease. 2013;**10**:944-950

[53] Takeshita M, Ishida Y, Akamatsu E, Ohmori Y, Sudoh M, Uto H, et al. Proanthocyanidin from blueberry leavessuppresses expression of subgenomic hepatitis C virus RNA. The Journal of Biological Chemistry. 2009;**284**:21165-21176

[54] Ali BH, Al Wabel N, Blunden G. Phytochemical, pharmacological and toxicological aspects of *Hibiscus sabdariffa* L.: A review. Phytotherapy Research. 2005;**19**(5):369-375

[55] Morton J. Roselle. In: Fruits of Warm Climates. Miami, FL: Creative Resource Systems Inc.; 1987. pp. 281-286

[56] Tsai P-J, McIntosh J, Pearce P, Camden B, Jordan BR. Anthocyanin and antioxidant capacity in Roselle (*Hibiscus sabdariffa* L.) extract. Food Research International. 2002;**35**(4):351-356

[57] Lin HH, Huang HP, Huang CC, Chen JH, Wang CJ. Hibiscus polyphenol-rich extract induces apoptosis inhuman gastric carcinoma cells via p53 phosphorylation and p38MAPK/FasL cascade pathway. Molecular Carcinogenesis. 2005;**43**(2):86-99

[58] McKay DL, Chen CY, Saltzman E, Blumberg JB. *Hibiscus sabdariffa* L. tea (tisane) lowers blood pressure in prehypertensive and mildly hypertensive adults. Journal of Nutrition. 2010;**140**(2):298-303

[59] Yang YS, Wang CJ, Huang CN, Chen ML, Chen MJ, Peng CH. Polyphenols of *Hibiscus sabdariffa* improved diabetic nephropathy via attenuating renal epithelial mesenchymal transition. Journal of Agriculture and Food Chemistry. 2013;**61**(31):7545-7551

[60] Liu KS, Tsao SM, Yin MC. In vitro antibacterial activity of roselle calyx and protocatechuic acid. Phytotherapy Research. 2005;**19**(11):942-945

[61] Borges A, Ferreira C, Saavedra MJ, Simoes M. Antibacterial activity and mode of action of ferulic and gallicacids against pathogenic bacteria. Microbial Drug Resistance. 2013;**19**(4):256-265

[62] Saini P, Gayen P, Nayak A, Kumar D, Mukherjee N, Pal BC, et al. Effect of ferulic acid from *Hibiscus mutabilis* onfilarial parasite *Setaria cervi*: Molecular and biochemical approaches. Parasitology International. 2012;**61**(4):520-531

[63] Kassem AF, Shaheen MNF, Batran RZ, Abbas EMH, Elseginy SA, Elmahdy EM. New 4-phenylcoumarin derivatives as potent 3C protease inhibitors: Design, synthesis, anti-HAV effect and molecular modeling. European Journal of Medicinal Chemistry. 2019;**168**:447-460

[64] Batran RZ, Kassem AF, Abbas EMH, Elseginy SA, Mounier MM. Design, synthesis and molecular modeling of new 4-phenylcoumarin derivatives astubulin polymerization inhibitors targeting MCF-7 breast cancer cells. Bioorganic and Medicinal Chemistry. 2018;**26**:3474-3490

[65] Garro HA, Pungitore CR. Coumarins as potential inhibitors of DNA polymerases and reverse transcriptases. Searching new antiretroviral and antitumoral drugs. Current Drug Discovery Technologies. 2015;**12**:66-79

[66] Bedoya LM, Beltran M, Sancho R, Olmedo DA, Sanchez-Palomino S, del Olmo E, et al. 4-Phenylcoumarins as HIV transcription inhibitors. Bioorganic & Medicinal Chemistry Letters. 2005;**15**:4447-4450

[67] Marquez N, Sancho R, Bedoya LM, Alcamí J, Lopez-Perez JL, Feliciano AS, et al. Mesuol, a natural occurring 4-phenylcoumarin, inhibits HIV-1 replication by targeting the NF-kappa B pathway. Antiviral Research. 2005;**66**:137-145

[68] Gill TA, Singer DS, Thompson JW. Purification and analysis of protamine. Process Biochemistry. 2006;**41**:1875-1882

[69] Islam NMD, Oda H, Motohiro T. Changes in the cell morphology and the release of soluble constituents from washed cells of *Bacillus subtillis* by the action of protamine. Nippon Suisan Gakkaishi. 1987;**53**:297-303

[70] Behçet A. The source-synthesis-history and use of atropine. The Journal of Academic Emergency Medicine. 2014;**13**:2-3

[71] Win NN, Kanda T, Nakamoto S, Moriyama M, Jiang X, Suganami A, et al. Inhibitory effect of Japanese rice-koji miso extracts on hepatitis A virus replication in association with the elevation of glucose-regulated protein 78 expression. International Journal of Medical Sciences. 2018;**15**(11):1153-1159

[72] Jiang X, Ren Q, Chen SP, et al. UVC mutagenicity is suppressed in Japanese miso-treated human RSa cells, possibly via GRP78 expression. Bioscience, Biotechnology, and Biochemistry. 2011;**75**:1685-1691

[73] Jiang X, Kanda T, Haga Y, et al. Glucose-regulated protein 78 is an antiviral against hepatitis A virus replication. Experimental and Therapeutic Medicine. 2017;**13**:3305-3308

[74] Park SY, Ha S-D. Inactivation of murine norovirus-1 and hepatitis A virus in the Korean traditional preserved raw crab product Ganjanggejang by soy sauce during storage. Food Control. 2015;**51**:293-299

[75] Choi NS, Chung SJ, Choi JY, Kim HW, Cho JJ. Physico-chemical and sensory properties of commercial Korean Traditional Soy sauce of mass produced vs. small scale farm produced in the Gyeonggi area. The Korean Journal of Food and Nutrition. 2013;**26**:553-564

[76] Masuda S, Hara-Kudo Y, Kumagai S. Reduction of *Escherichia coli* O157:H7 populations in soy sauce, a fermented seasoning. Journal of Food Protection. 1998;**61**:657-661

[77] Kim JS, Moon GS, Lee YS. Chromaticity and brown pigment patterns of soy sauce and UHYUKJANG, Korean traditional fermented soy sauce. Korean Journal of Food and Cookery Science. 1996;**23**:642-649

[78] Mao S, Wang M, Ou X, Sun D, Cheng A, Zhu D, et al. Virologic and immunologic characteristics in mature ducks with acute duck hepatitis A virus 1 infection. Frontiers in Immunology. 2017;**8**:1574

[79] Song M, Chen Y, Du H, Zhang S, Wang Y, Zeng L, et al. Raw Rehmannia radix polysaccharide can effectively release peroxidative injury induced by duck hepatitis A virus. African Journal of Traditional, Complementary, and Alternative Medicines. 2017;**14**(4):8-21

[80] Ming K, Chen Y, Yao F, Shi J, Yang J, Du H, et al. Phosphorylated *Codonopsis pilosula* polysaccharide could inhibit the virulence of duck hepatitis A virus compared with *Codonopsis pilosula* polysaccharide. International Journal of Biological Macromolecules. 2017;**94**:28-35

[81] Chen Y, Yang Y, Wang F, Yang X, Yao F, Ming K, et al. Antiviral effect of baicalin phospholipid complex against duck hepatitis Avirus type 1. Poultry Science. 2018;**97**(8):2722-2732

[82] Chen Y, Zeng L, Lu Y, Yang Y, Xu M, Wang Y, et al. Treatment effect of a flavonoid prescription on duck virus hepatitis by its hepatoprotective and antioxidative ability. Pharmaceutical Biology. 2017;**55**(1):198-205

Section 3

Other Hepatobiliary Conditions

Chapter 7

Hepatic Involvement in Hemophagocytic Lymphohistiocytosis

Somanath Padhi, RajLaxmi Sarangi, Susama Patra and Subash Chandra Samal

Abstract

Hemophagocytic lymphohistiocytosis (HLH) is a hyperinflammatory syndrome which results in uncontrolled systemic proliferation of benign macrophages in all reticuloendothelial organs producing worsening peripheral blood cytopenia(s); hypercytokinemia leading to hepatic injury producing hyperferritinemia, hypertriglyceridemia, hypofibrinogenemia; and if not diagnosed and treated early may lead to disseminated intravascular coagulation (DIC), multiorgan dysfunction, and death in nearly all individuals. It is postulated that hepatic injury/dysfunction starts early in the course of the disease which may mimic nonspecific hepatitis like prodrome to fulminant hepatic failure; possibly requiring liver transplant. While HLH as an entity is being increasingly recognized nowadays across wide specialties (both pediatric and adults); hepatic involvement in this setting has been poorly characterized. This chapter is aimed to highlight on the diagnosis and classification of HLH with a special emphasis on the pathophysiology of hepatic dysfunction, histomorphology of liver; and the current concept and controversies on the role of liver transplantation in this clinical setting.

Keywords: cytokine storm, HLH, liver, transplant, outcome

1. Introduction

Hemophagocytic lymphohistiocytosis (HLH) or hemophagocytic syndrome is a potentially catastrophic hyperinflammatory syndrome occurring in genetically susceptible individuals which results due to hyperactive, yet inappropriate, immune system going runamock [1]. This results due to impaired cytotoxic T lymphocyte (CTL)/natural killer (NK) cell activity producing uncontrolled proliferation of benign macrophages in all reticuloendothelial organs such as bone marrow, spleen, liver, and lymph nodes; causing histiocytic hemophagocytosis, worsening unexplained peripheral blood cytopenia (s), cytokine storm, cytokine mediated hepatic injury/dysfunction producing spectrum of biochemical alteration such as hyperferritinemia, hypertriglyceridemia, hypofibrinogenemia, coagulopathy, disseminated intravascular coagulation (DIC), multi organ dysfunction (MOD); and if not diagnosed and treated early, may lead to death in virtually all case [2]. Since the first description of cases coined as "histiocytic medullary reticulocytosis" by Scott Robin and Smith in 1939, there has been a sequential change in nomenclature of this entity [3–6]. While HLH

IntechOpen

as an entity is being increasingly recognized nowadays across wide specialties (both pediatric and adults); hepatic involvement in this setting has been poorly characterized [7–9]. Hepatomegaly and hepatic dysfunction, including elevated serum transaminases and bilirubin, cholestasis, and coagulopathy typically occur early in the disease and are associated with marked hematologic and/or neurological abnormalities. In rare instances acute hepatic failure may dominate the clinical picture, which in combination with hyperferritinemia, may mimic neonatal hemochromatosis [10].

2. Classification of HLH

Traditionally, HLH has been broadly classified into two forms: (i) primary HLH which is known to harbor documented genetic abnormalities implicated in the cytotoxic functions of the NK cell/CTL; and (ii) a secondary form which occurs in adults/elderly population without any genetic abnormality. However, upon the realization that HLH defining genetic abnormality can occur in any age, that these defects may be uncommon even in pediatric age group, the designations *primary and secondary* have become less relevant; and stratification into *genetic and acquired* forms seems more appropriate [11]. The genetic variant is again subdivided into autosomal recessive familial HLH (FHL) involving the several mutations in the CTL/NK

Type	Examples with proportions in parentheses
A. Genetic	
i. Autosomal recessive/familial HLH	PFR1/perforin 1 (20-50%), UNC13D/Munc 13-4 (20%), STX11/syntaxin 11 (1%), STXB2/syntaxin binding protein 2 or UNC18B (unknown)
ii. Associated with primary immunodeficiency syndromes	Chediak-Higashi syndrome (LYST), Griscelli syndrome type 2 (RAB27A/Rab27a), Hermansky-Pudlak syndrome type 2 (AP3B1), X-linked proliferative syndrome (XLP) type 1 (SHD2D1A/SAP protein), X-linked proliferative syndrome (XLP) type 2 (BIRC4/XIAP protein)
B.Acquired	
i. Virus associated	Herpes viruses (EBV, CMV, HHV-8, HSV), HIV, HTLV, adenovirus, HAV, HBV, HCV, measles, mumps, rubella, dengue, hantavirus, parvovirus B19, Enterovirus, influenza
ii. Bacteria associated	*Staphylococcus aureus*, *Campylobacter* spp., *Fusobacterium* spp., *Mycoplasma* spp., *Chlamydia* spp., *Legionella* spp., *Salmonella typhi*, *Rickettsia* spp., *Brucella* spp., *Ehrlichia* spp., *Borrelia burgdorferi*, *Mycobacterium tuberculosis*
iii. Fungal associated	*Candida* spp., *Cryptococcus* spp., *Pneumocystis* spp., *Histoplasma* spp., *Aspergillus* spp., *Fusarium* spp.
iv. Parasitic	*Plasmodium falciparum*, *Plasmodium vivax*, *Toxoplasma* spp., *Babesia* spp., *Strongyloides* spp., *Leishmania* spp.
v. Malignancy associated	Peripheral T-cell/NK-cell lymphomas, ALCL, ALL, Hodgkin lymphoma, multiple myeloma, acute erythroid leukemia Prostate and lung cancer, hepatocellular carcinoma
vi. Autoimmune disease associated (macrophage activation syndrome, MAS)	Systemic-onset juvenile idiopathic arthritis, Kawasaki disease, systemic lupus erythematosus, seronegative spondyloarthropathies

Table 1.
Classification of hemophagocytic lymphohistiocytosis (HLH) (adopted from Rosado et al. [1] and Gholam et al. [12]).

cell cytotoxic pathways [PFR1/perforin 1 (20–50%), UNC13D/Munc 13-4 (20%), STX11/syntaxin 11 (1%), STXB2/syntaxin binding protein 2 or UNC18B (unknown)] and those associated with primary immunodeficiency syndromes such as Chédiak-Higashi syndrome (LYST), Griscelli syndrome type 2 (RAB27A/Rab27a), Hermansky-Pudlak syndrome type 2 (AP3B1), and X-linked proliferative syndrome (XLP) type 1 (SHD2D1A/SAP protein) and type 2 (BIRC4/XIAP protein) [12] (**Table 1**).

Acquired form of HLH is known to be triggered by diverse etiologies in susceptible individuals; and are segregated as (i) infection associated secondary to viruses (notably EVB, CMV, HHV-8, HSV, dengue, parvo B19, HAV, HBV, HCV, etc.; any bacteria, fungi, parasites such as Plasmodia, Leishmania, Strongyloides), (ii) malignancy associated (NK-T cell lymphoma/leukemia, anaplastic large cell lymphoma, plasma cell myeloma, Hodgkin lymphoma, B cell non Hodgkin lymphoma, acute lymphoid and myeloid leukemias; and solid malignancies such as lung cancer, hepatocellular carcinoma, etc.), and (iii) macrophage activation syndrome or MAS (associated with autoimmune disorders) [1, 3, 13].

3. Diagnostic criteria

There has been a paradigm shift of focus in the diagnosis of HLH since 2004 (**Table 2**) [3]. The 2004 diagnostic criteria developed for the pediatric HLH have been widely adopted in adult medicine without systematic validation. Both 2004 and 2009 guidelines incorporated mutational/genetic analysis as a "major criterion" which has subsequently been taken out, especially for adult HLH case. Moreover, two important parameters that were incorporated in previous criteria such as "impaired NK cell activity" and "increased soluble interleukin 2 receptor" are likely to be removed sooner or later as these tests are available in only very few specialized centers all over the world and are very costly. Therefore, in practice, the necessary five out of eight criteria as per the HLH 2004 guidelines are actually five out of six parameters tested. In addition, the criteria of "bone marrow hemophagocytosis" is becoming increasingly less important nowadays as histiocytic hemophagocytosis has a poor specificity in the diagnosis of HLH and this may not even be evident during initial marrow evaluation [1]! In order to overcome these shortcomings, the French investigators proposed to adopt a new objective scoring system (HLH probability score or HScore) (**Table 3**). A total probability score of 169 was found to have a higher sensitivity and specificity for the diagnosis of HLH [6]. Furthermore, simpler routine laboratory parameters (extended variables) have been incorporated to diagnose the disease early. These include peripheral blood monocytosis, hyponatremia, elevated lactate dehydrogenase, elevated β2 microglobulin, impaired coagulation parameters, and CSF pleocytosis [14].

Another interesting change has been made in regard to the measurement of serum ferritin. A ≥ 500 μg/L cut off among pediatric population (up to 18 years of age) was found to have 84% sensitivity in HLH-1994 trial and therefore was included in the HLH 2004 guidelines [15]. Subsequently, pediatricians have revised their ferritin cut off value to ≥10,000 μg/L with a higher sensitivity and near 100% specificity for the diagnosis of HLH [16]. On the contrary, recent reports from adult intensive care units (ICUs) have suggested a lower ferritin cut off value of 3000 to 4000 μg/L with >80% sensitivity and specificity in HLH diagnosis [17]. While hyperferritinemia is not specific to HLH, the same in the clinical context of fever, worsening cytopenia (s), and splenomegaly is highly valuable in the ICUs where sepsis is the major overlapping clinical condition [18]. Recent studies have shown that a high serum soluble interleukin 2 receptor to ferritin ratio is an important biomarker in distinguishing lymphoma associated HLH compared to benign disease associated HLH (8.56 vs. 0.66, respectively, $P = 0.0004$) [19].

Diagnostic parameters	HLH diagnostic criteria					
	HLH-1994	HLH-1997	HLH-2004	HLH-2009	HLH-2014	HLH-2016
Molecular diagnosis	x	x	√	√	x	x
Immunosuppression (**Table 3**)	x	x	x	x	√	x
Fever	√	√	√	√	√	√
Splenomegaly	√	√	√	√	√	√
Cytopenia (s)¶	√	√	√	√	√	√
Hyperferritinemia¶¶	x	x	√	√	√	√
Hypertriglyceridemia¶¶¶	√	√	√	√	√	√
Hypofibrinogenemia≠	√	√	√	√	√	√
Hemophagocytosis	√	√	√	√	√	√§
Decreased NK cell activity§§	x	x	√	√	x	x
Increased soluble IL2 receptor§§	x	x	√	√	x	x
Raised SGOT	x	x	x	x	√	x
Required number of criteria	All	All	5/8 or molecular diagnosis	2 major or 1 major and 4 minors	HScore (probability score) (**Table-3**)	
Supportive featuresǀ	x	x	x	x	√	√

¶Hemoglobin; <90 g/L (in infants <4 weeks old, <100 g/L); Platelets $<100 \times 10^9/L$; Neutrophils $<1.0 \times 10^9/L$).
¶¶≥ 500 µg/L.
¶¶¶Fasting triglycerides ≥3.0 mmol/L (≥265 mg/dL).
≠≤1.5 g/L.
§In bone marrow aspirate.
§§Likely to be dropped as a criteria.
ǀCoagulopathy, hyperbilirubinemia, hypoalbuminemia, hyponatremia, raised lactate dehydrogenase, elevated β2 microglobulin, peripheral blood monocytosis, CSF pleocytosis, etc.
√ Included in the criteria. x Not included in the criteria.

Table 2.
Updated diagnostic criteria for HLH [3–6, 14].

4. Pathophysiology of HLH

Genetic HLH results due to inability to clear the antigenic stimulus and thus turn off the inflammatory response is what ultimately leads to *cytokine storm* characteristic of HLH. In healthy individuals, viral and tumor antigenic stimuli leads to Th1 mediated cytokine response (IFN-γ, TNF-α, GM-CSF) which in turn, stimulates CTL and NK cells to clear off target cells (viral infected cells, tumor cells, etc.) through release of perforin and granzyme granules at the synaptic site. Perforin is a key cytolytic protein that acts by inserting itself in the membrane of the target cell and creating pores that lead to osmotic lysis of the target cell. The normal production of vesicle granule content requires orchestrated steps of maturation, polarization, docking, fusion, and finally degranulation in the immunological synapse. All the genetic defects described in FHL involve either inadequate levels of perforin itself (FHL2) or improper granule exocytosis (FHL3–5 and immunodeficiency syndromes) (see above in the classification) (**Figure 1**) [2, 20].

Parameters	Number of points (criteria for scoring)
Known immunosuppression¶	0 (no) or 18 (yes)
Temperature (°C)	0 (<38.4), 33 (38.4-39.4), or 49 (>39.4)
Organomegaly	0 (no), 23 (hepatomegaly or splenomegaly), or 38 (hepatomegaly and splenomegaly
Number of cytopenia (s)‡	0 (1 lineage), 24 (2 lineages), or 34 (3 lineages)
Ferritin (μg/L)	0 (< 2000), 35 (2000–6000), or 50 (>6000)
Triglyceride (mmoles/L)	0 (<1.5), 44 (1.5–4), or 64 (>4)
Fibrinogen (g/L)	0 (>2.5), or 30 (≤ 2.5)
Serum SGOT (IU/L)	0 (< 30), or 19 (≥ 30)
Hemophagocytosis in marrow aspirate	0 (no) or 35 (yes)

¶Human immunodeficiency virus or receiving long term immunosuppressive therapy (glucocorticoids, cyclosporine, azathioprine).
‡Hb ≤ 92 g/L, total leukocyte count ≤ 5000/mm^3, platelet count ≤ 110,000/mm^3.

Table 3.
Hemophagocytic lymphohistiocytosis probability score (HScore) as proposed by Fardet et al. [6].

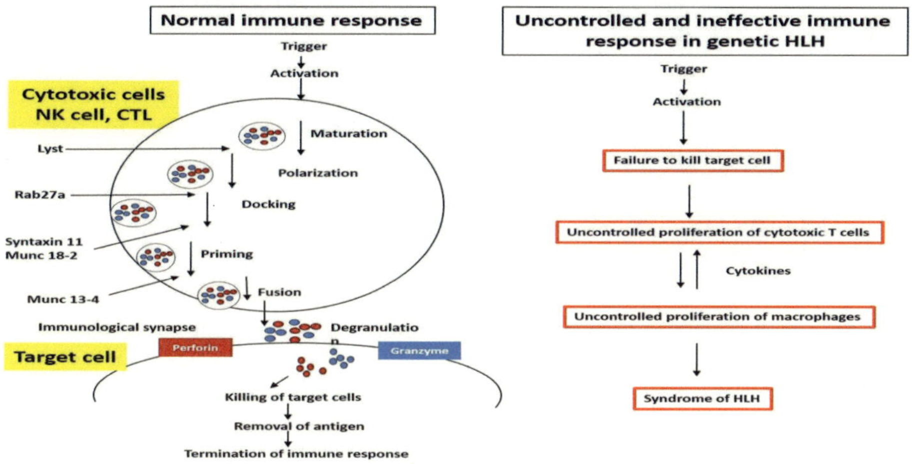

Figure 1.
Immune response in healthy subjects and uncontrolled, ineffective immune response in patients with genetic HLH. Adopted and modified from Janka GE [2].

5. Pathophysiology of hepatic dysfunction: the cytokine theory

It is now postulated that hepatic injury/dysfunction HLH is mainly due to cytokine storm which results due to impaired NK/Cytotoxic T lymphocyte function in a *genetically susceptible* individual while triggering factors playing a crucial role. The up regulation of granulocytic monocytic colony stimulating factor receptor on the macrophages along with macrophage proliferation leads to splenohepatomegaly. The macrophage derived IL-2, IFN-γ, and TNF-α mediated inflammation is reported to be predominantly porto-sinusoidal rather than lobular without any significant alteration in lobular architecture; which in turn produces raised transaminases, hepatocyte hemosiderosis; sinusoidal dilatation and congestion, Kupffer cell hyperplasia and hypertrophy producing hemosiderosis and hemophagocytosis. Furthermore, lymphocyte or lymphohistiocyte mediated biliary ductular injury

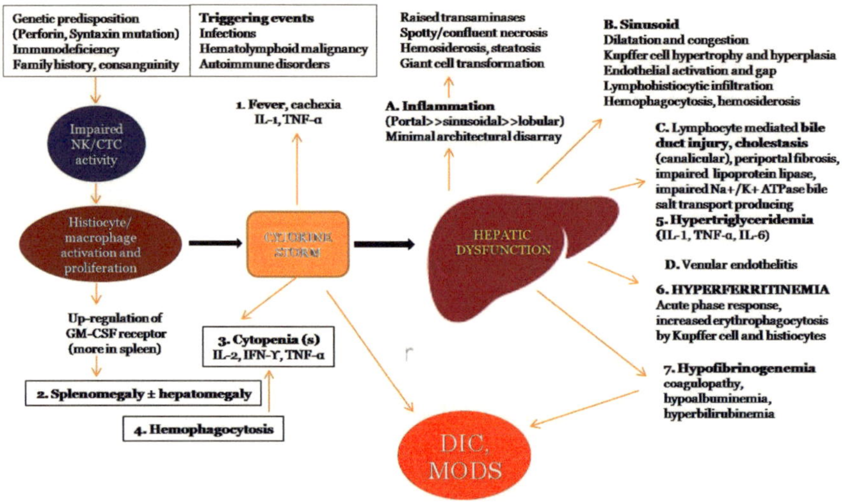

Figure 2.
Cytokine basis of HLH associated hepatic dysfunction. GM-CSF; granulocytic monocytic colony stimulating factor, IL; interleukin, IFN-γ; interferon gamma, TNF-α; tumor necrosis factor alpha, DIC; disseminated intravascular coagulation, MODS; multiorgan dysfunction syndrome. Note the parameters from no. 1 to 7 are incorporated in the HLH criteria. The pathophysiologic features assigned A to D are related to cytokine mediated liver parenchymal alteration (see below). Schematic representation summarized from de Kerguenec et al. [9] and Billiau et al. [21].

and cytokine (IL 1, IL 6, and TNF-α) mediated impaired lipoprotein lipase activity causes cholestasis, hyperbilirubinemia and hypertriglyceridemia. Finally, hyperferritinemia so characteristic of HLH, is nothing but the result of acute phase reaction as well as increased erythrophagocytosis by Kupffer cells. All these cytokine basis of hepatic injury may culminate in severe hepatic functional compromise leading to hypofibrinogenemia, hypoalbuminemia, disseminated intravascular coagulation, and multiorgan dysfunction with a fatal outcome (**Figure 2**).

6. Histology of liver in HLH

The morphology of liver in HLH is not well characterized because of insufficient biopsy data, late diagnosis, sampling bias (needle biopsy vs. wedge biopsy); and associated triggering factors such as virus associated histological alterations; especially in acquired cases (**Table 4**).

Morphological changes as observed in several large series of liver biopsy specimens have shown relatively well-preserved hepatic parenchyma with a portal and sinusoidal lymphohistiocytic, CD 3+, CD8+, Granzyme B+, and variable perforin+ T cell-rich infiltrate [7–9, 21, 22]. Diverse histological patterns have been described in such cases (**Table 4**): (i) adult type *chronic hepatitis* like characterized by *mild* portal lymphocytic infiltrate with mild bile duct injury and endothelialitis, reported to be so *characteristic* of neonatal/childhood HLH; (ii) *leukemia like* pattern characterized by *extensive* portal, lymphohistiocytic infiltrate expanding the tracts and encroaching upon the lobular periphery blurring the portal limiting plate and infiltrating the sinusoids; (iii) *histiocytic storage disorder-like* pattern characterized by massive infiltration of histiocyte rich infiltrate plugging and distending the sinusoids and venules; (iv) *neonatal giant cell hepatitis-like* pattern characterized by extensive giant cell transformation of hepatocytes with prominent *architectural disarray*; (v) increased hepatic hemosiderosis along with marked hyperferritinemia and features of acute liver failure mimicking *neonatal hemochromatosis*; (vi) post stem cell transplantation *graft*

Sl.no, age, gender	C/F as per HLH-2004	Architecture disarray (present/absent); Inflammation: location, nature, Pattern, necrosis, hemosiderosis	Cholestasis/ steatosis	Lymphocyte mediated bile duct injury; nature of inflammation	Sinusoid(dilatation/ inflammation	Kupffer cell (number/ hemosiderosis	Hp	Venules (endothelialitis)	Outcome
1. 12d, M	All	Present; Severe, lobular >> portal, *Giant cell hepatitis like*, spotty necrosis	++/x	++; *Giant cell hepatitis like*; CD8/ Gr. B/Perforin+ T cell	Yes/LH type	↑/x	+++	Yes	Death
2. 7m, M	All	Absent; Moderate to severe, centrilobular hepatitis, *chronic active GVHD*	++/x	+, fibrosis, Perforin+ T cells	Yes/lymphocytic	↑/+	Mild	No	Death
3. 16d, M	All	Present; lobular >> portal, *Giant cell hepatitis like*, increased iron in hepatocytes (+++) *mimicking neonatal hemochromatosis*	++/x	++, *Giant cell hepatitis like*; CD8+/Perforin− T cells	Yes/LH type	↑/+++	+++	Yes	Death
4. 25d, -	ALF	Absent; Portal >> lobules; centrilobular necrosis	+++	+++, *leukemia like,* CD8/Gr. B/ Perforin+	Yes/dense lymphocytic	↑/x	+++	Yes, Congestion	
5. 2m, M	ARF	Absent; Portal >> lobules	+/++	+++; *chronic persistent hepatitis like*, CD8/Gr B/ Perforin+ T cells	Yes/lymphocytic	↑/+	+++	Yes	Death
6.2m, F	All	Absent; Portal >> lobules	+/++	+++; *leukemia like;* Perforin+ T cells	Yes/LH type	↑/+	++	Yes	Alive

Sl.no, age, gender	C/F as per HLH-2004	Architecture disarray (present/absent); Inflammation: location, nature, Pattern, necrosis, hemosiderosis	Cholestasis/ steatosis	Lymphocyte mediated bile duct injury; nature of inflammation	Sinusoid(dilatation/ inflammation	Kupffer cell (number/ hemosiderosis	Hp	Venules (endothelialitis)	Outcome
7. 2m, M	All	Absent; Portal >> lobules, hemosiderosis (+)	++/x	+++; *leukemia like;* CD8/Gr B/ Perforin+ T cells	Yes/LH type	↑/+	+	Yes	Death
8. 3m, M	All	Absent; lobular >> portal, *chronic hepatitis like*	+++/+	+; *chronic persistent hepatitis like*; CD8/ Gr B+/Perforin– T cells	Yes/LH type	↑/++	+	Yes	Death
9. 3m, M	ALF	Absent; Portal>>lobular, hepatic siderosis (+++)	++/+	+++, *leukemia like*, CD8/Gr B+/ Perforin+ T cells	Yes/leukemia like	↑/+	+++	Yes	Death
10. 3m, M	Sibling	Absent; Portal>>lobular	++/x	+++, *leukemia like,* CD8/Gr B+/ Perforin+ T cells	Yes/LH type	↑/x	+++	ND	Death
11. 3m, M	All	Present, Lobular>>portal; *Giant cell hepatitis*	+/+	++, CD8/Gr B+/ Perforin+ T cells	Yes/LH type	↑/x	+++	Yes	Death
12. 3m, F	All	Present; Portal>>lobular; *Giant cell hepatitis like pattern*	+/+	++, *chronic persistent hepatitis like* CD8/Gr B+/ Perforin+ T cells	Yes/LH type	↑/x	+++	Yes	
13. 3m, M	All, consanguinity	Absent; Portal>>lobular	+/x	+++, *Leukemia like*, CD8/Gr B+/ Perforin+ T cells	Yes/LH type	↑/x	+++	Yes	Death

Sl.no, age, gender	C/F as per HLH-2004	Architecture disarray (present/absent); Inflammation: location, nature, Pattern, necrosis, hemosiderosis	Cholestasis/ steatosis	Lymphocyte mediated bile duct injury; nature of inflammation	Sinusoid(dilatation/ inflammation	Kupffer cell (number/ hemosiderosis	Hp	Venules (endothelialitis)	Outcome
14. 3m, M	All	Absent; Portal>>lobular; *chronic hepatitis like*	+/x	++, *chronic persistent hepatitis like*, CD8/Gr B+/ Perforin+ T cells	Yes/LH type	↑/x	+++	Yes	Death
15. 4m, M	Sibling	Absent, Portal>>lobular; chronic hepatitis like	+/x	+++, *Leukemia like*, CD8/Gr B+/ Perforin+ T cells	Yes/LH type	↑/x	+++	Yes	Death
16. 8m, F	ALF	Absent, centrilobular hemorrhage, atrophy of hepatic cords	++/++	++, *Storage histiocytic like*, CD8/Gr B+/ Perforin+ T cells, perivenous fibrosis	Yes/histiocytic infiltrate like storage cells	↑/++	+++	Yes	Death
17. 8m, M	All, HCV positive	Absent, portal>>lobular, hepatic hemosiderosis (+++)	++/+	+++; *leukemia like*, CD8/Gr B+/ Perforin+ T cells	Yes/LH type	↑/++	+++	Yes	Lost to follow-up
18. 9m, M	All	Absent, portal>>lobular	+/+	++; *chronic persistent hepatitis like*, CD8/Gr B+/ Perforin+ T cells	Yes/LH type	↑/++	+++	Yes	Death
19. 11m, F	All	Absent, portal>>lobular	++/++	+++; *leukemia like*, CD8/Gr B+/ Perforin+ T cells	Yes/LH type	↑/+	+++	Yes	Death

Sl.no, age, gender	**C/F as per HLH-2004**	**Architecture disarray (present/absent); Inflammation: location, nature, Pattern, necrosis, hemosiderosis**	**Cholestasis/ steatosis**	**Lymphocyte mediated bile duct injury; nature of inflammation**	**Sinusoid(dilatation/ inflammation**	**Kupffer cell (number/ hemosiderosis**	**Hp**	**Venules (endothelialitis)**	**Outcome**
27. children	1^0HLH (11 M, 16 F)	Absent; portal >>> lobular	Not described	++ to +++, *chronic persistent hepatitis like (characteristic)*	Yes/LH type	↑/x	+	Not studied	Autopsy series [8]
30. adults	2^0HLH (19 M, 11 F) ALF like in 19/29	Absent; portal >>> lobular; hepatocyte necrosis (focal in 10; diffuse in 4), siderosis in 11	++/++	++ to +++; LH type to tumoral infiltration, no ductular proliferation or damage or ductopenia, *no Hp in portal area*	Yes/LH type, erythrophagocytosis	↑/++	++/+++	Not described	Ref. [9]

Footnotes: d; days, m; months, M; male, F; female, C/F; clinical feature, ALF; acute liver failure, ARF; acute renal failure, GVHD; graft versus host disease, +; mild/inconspicuous, ++; moderate, +++; marked, x; not present, Gr. B; granzyme B, LH; lymphohistiocytic, ↑; increase in number, ND; not described, Hp; hemophagocytosis.

Table 4.
Histopathology of liver in cases with hemophagocytic lymphohistiocytosis as described in several series (Chen et al. [10], n = 19; Ost et al. [8], n = 27; de Kerguenec et al. [9], n = 30).

versus host disease related changes; (vii) *lymphocyte depleted* morphology unrelated to prior immunosuppressive or immunomodulator therapy; especially later in the course of the disease or as a part of aberrant cytokine modulation [10].

Common to all specimens and helpful in diagnosing HLH are a constellation of *additional* features that included distinctive lymphocyte-mediated bile duct injury, significant endothelialitis of terminal portal and central veins, sinusoidal congestion and dilatation, increased Kupffer cell activity with or without hemosiderosis, erythrophagocytosis, and histiocytic hemophagocytosis which is reported as inconspicuous to florid. Steatosis and cholestasis were also usually present [8–10]. The *lymphocyte-mediated bile duct injury* is characterized by nests or circumferential sheaths of lymphomononuclear cells interposed between the epithelium and the basal lamina eliciting *little damage* to the epithelium. The portal inflammation with cholangitis observed in FHL is reminiscent of primary sclerosing cholangitis, primary biliary cirrhosis, and vanishing bile duct syndrome; though neutrophils, plasma cells, granulomatous inflammation, periductal sclerosis, or ductopenia common in latter conditions are reported to be rare in HLH cases [10]. *Endothelialitis* of terminal hepatic and portal veins may result in transmural phlebitis and hemorrhage and extensive apoptosis of perivenular hepatocytes. The degree of inflammation, bile duct damage, endothelialitis, cholestasis, and steatosis seem to reflect the clinical stage of the disease.

7. Liver transplantation: current concept and controversies

The mortality rate is very high in HLH associated acute liver failure cases. However, this association is extremely rare. Moreover, the presence of two clinical conditions (HLH and acute liver failure) together makes its further complicated and delays the diagnosis. The average time from earliest diagnosis of liver failure to a definitive diagnosis of HLH has been reported to be 17.27 days [23]. This suggests that HLH is a late occurring phenomenon in the process of ALF. On the contrary, there are reports which support the viewpoint of HLH causing liver injury and thus culminating in ALF [24, 25]. The exact mechanism is still not known, as far as HLH induced liver injury is concerned. It is most probably the infiltration of activated macrophage or over production of cytokine in HLH can explain the degree of liver injury. In a clinical scenario, where the patient present with prolonged fever, jaundice and pancytopenia; HLH should be considered as a differential diagnosis [23]. The role of liver transplantation in the treatment of HLH – ALF is controversial. It is so, because of the primarily systemic nature of the disease, the risk of hepatic recurrence of HLH during the post-transplant period, increased in rejection rate and poor general condition of the patient to tolerate the transplant procedure [26]. The post-transplant survival at the end of 6 months is only 33% for the primary HLH – ALF patient [27]. However, a small clinical series involving nine pediatric patients, reported a better survival rate among the secondary HLH – ALF group [26].

In the secondary form of HLH, the liver transplantation is also not very helpful in the situation such as absence of ALF (MELD score < 20–22); when the clinical severity is due to the combined effect of ALF and HLH, rather than ALF alone; and when the HLH is severe and highly likely to be irreversible. In these situations, high mortality from advanced and likely irreversible HLH may limit the benefits of liver transplantation [28]. Liver biopsy should be performed to decide the extent of the liver injury and the role played by the hepatic injury vs. systemic HLH in the patients with ALF. However, liver transplant is still an option in HLH – ALF cases with predominant liver involvement from HLH and this should be undertaken before the highly lethal complication of HLH, such as, septic shock, DIC, bone marrow failure, explosive immune activation from HLH supervenes.

Author details

Somanath Padhi[1]*, RajLaxmi Sarangi[2], Susama Patra[1] and Subash Chandra Samal[3]

1 Department of Pathology with Laboratory Medicine, All India Institute of Medical Sciences, Bhubaneswar, India

2 Department of Biochemistry, Kalinga Institute of Medical Sciences, Bhubaneswar, India

3 Department of Gastroenterology, All India Institute of Medical Sciences, Bhubaneswar, India

*Address all correspondence to: pathol_somanath@aiimsbhubaneswar.edu.in

References

[1] Rosado FGN, Kim AS. Hemophagocytic lymphohistiocytosis: An update on diagnosis and pathogenesis. American Journal of Clinical Pathology. 2013;**139**:713727. DOI: 10.1309/AJCP4ZDKJ4ICOUAT

[2] Janka GE. Familial and acquired hemophagocytic lymphohistiocytosis. Annual Review of Medicine. 2012;**63**:233-246. DOI: 10.1146/annurev-med-041610-134208

[3] Hayden A, Park S, Giustini D, Lee AY, Chen LY. Hemophagocytic syndromes (HPSs) including hemophagocytic lymphohistiocytosis (HLH) in adults: A systematic scoping review. Blood Reviews. 2016;**30**:411-420. DOI: 10.1016/j.blre.2016.05.001

[4] Henter JI, Horne A, Aricó M, Egeler RM, Filipovich AH, Imashuku S, et al. HLH-2004: Diagnostic and therapeutic guidelines for hemophagocytic lymphohistiocytosis. Pediatric Blood & Cancer. 2007;**48**:124-131. DOI: 10.1002/pbc.21039

[5] Filipovich AH. Hemophagocytic lymphohistiocytosis (HLH) and related disorders. Hematology. American Society of Hematology. Education Program. 2009;**2009**:127-131. DOI: 10.1182/asheducation-2009.1.127

[6] Fardet L, Galicier L, Lambotte O, Marzac C, Aumont C, Chahwan D, et al. Development and validation of the HScore, a score for the diagnosis of reactive hemophagocytic syndrome. Arthritis & Rhematology. 2014;**66**:2613-2620. DOI: 10.1002/art.38690

[7] Favara BE. Histopathology of the liver in histiocytosis syndromes. Pediatric Pathology & Laboratory Medicine. 1996;**16**:413-433. DOI: 10.1080/15513819609168681

[8] Ost A, Nilsson-Ardnor S, Henter JI. Autopsy findings in 27 children with haemophagocytic lymphohistiocytosis. Histopathology. 1998;**32**:310-316. DOI: 10.1046/j.1365-2559.1998.00377.x

[9] de Kerguenec C, Hillaire S, Molinié V, Gardin C, Degott C, Erlinger S, et al. Hepatic manifestations of hemophagocytic syndrome: A study of 30 cases. The American Journal of Gastroenterology. 2001;**96**:852-857. DOI: 10.1111/j.1572-0241.2001.03632.x

[10] Chen JH, Fleming MD, Pinkus GS, Pinkus JL, Nichols KE, Mo JQ, et al. Pathology of the liver in familial hemophagocytic lymphohistiocytosis. The American Journal of Surgical Pathology. 2010;**34**:852-867. DOI: 10.1097/PAS.0b013e3181dbbb17

[11] Janka GE, Lehmberg K. Hemophagocytic lymphohistiocytosis: Pathogenesis and treatment. Hematology. 2013;**2013**:605-611. DOI: 10.1182/asheducation-2013.1.605

[12] Gholam C, Grigoriadou S, Gilmour KC, Gaspar HB. Familial haemophagocytic lymphohistiocytosis: Advances in the genetic basis, diagnosis and management. Clinical and Experimental Immunology. 2011;**163**:271-283. DOI: 10.1111/j.1365-2249.2010.04302.x

[13] Padhi S, Varghese RG, Ramdas A, Phansalkar MD, Sarangi R. Hemophagocytic lymphohistiocytosis: Critical reappraisal of a potentially under-recognized condition. Frontiers in Medicine. 2013;**7**:492-498. DOI: 10.1007/s11684-013-0292-0

[14] Tamamyan GN, Kantarjian HM, Ning J, Jain P, Sasaki K, McClain KL, et al. Malignancy-associated hemophagocytic lymphohistiocytosis in adults: Relation to hemophagocytosis, characteristics, and outcomes. Cancer.

2016;**122**:2857-2866. DOI: 10.1002/cncr.30084

[15] Allen CE, Yu X, Kozinetz CA, McClain KL. Highly elevated ferritin levels and the diagnosis of hemophagocytic lymphohistiocytosis. Pediatric Blood & Cancer. 2008;**50**:1227-1235. DOI: 10.1002/pbc.21423

[16] Schram AM, Campigotto F, Mullally A, Fogerty A, Massarotti E, Neuberg D, et al. Marked hyperferritinemia does not predict for HLH in the adult population. Blood. 2015;**125**:1548-1552. DOI: 10.1182/blood-2014-10-602607

[17] Lachmann G, Spies C, Schenk T, Brunkhorst FM, Balzer F, La Rosée P, et al. Hemophagocytic lymphohistiocytosis: Potentially underdiagnosed in intensive care units. Shock. 2018;**50**:149-155. DOI: 10.1097/SHK.0000000000001048

[18] Sackett K, Cunderlik M, Sahni N, Killeen AA, Olson AP. Extreme hyperferritinemia: Causes and impact on diagnostic reasoning. American Journal of Clinical Pathology. 2016;**145**:646-650. DOI: 10.1093/ajcp/aqw053

[19] Tsuji T, Hirano T, Yamasaki H, Tsuji M, Tsuda H. A high sIL-2R/ferritin ratio is a useful marker for the diagnosis of lymphoma-associated hemophagocytic syndrome. Annals of Hematology. 2014;**93**:821-826. DOI: 10.1007/s00277-013-1925-8

[20] Janka G. Hemophagocytic lymphohistiocytosis: When the immune system runs amok. Klinische Pädiatrie. 2009;**22**:278-285. DOI: 10.1055/s-0029-1237386

[21] Billiau AD, Roskams T, Van Damme-Lombaerts R, Matthys P, Wouters C. Macrophage activation syndrome: Characteristic findings on liver biopsy illustrating the key role of activated, IFN-gamma-producing lymphocytes and IL-6- and TNF-alpha-producing macrophages. Blood. 2005;**105**:1648-1651. DOI: 10.1182/blood-2004-08-2997

[22] Kapelari K, Fruehwirth M, Heitger A, Königsrainer A, Margreiter R, Simma B, et al. Loss of intrahepatic bile ducts: An important feature of familial hemophagocytic lymphohistiocytosis. Virchows Archiv. 2005;**446**:619-625. DOI: 10.1007/s00428-005-1238-y

[23] Dong J, Xie F, Jia L, Li J, Hu Z, Zhu Y, et al. Clinical characteristics of liver failure with hemophagocytic lymphohistiocytosis. Scientific Reports. 2019;**9**:8125. DOI: 10.1038/s41598-019-43909-w

[24] Jagtap N, Sharma M, Rajesh G, Rao PN, Anuradha S, Tandan M, et al. Hemophagocytic lymphohistiocytosis masquerading as acute liver failure: A single center experience. Journal of Clinical and Experimental Hepatology. 2017;**7**:184-189. DOI: 10.1016/j.jceh.2017.01

[25] Lin S, Li Y, Long J, Liu Q, Yang F, He Y. Acute liver failure caused by hemophagocytic lymphohistiocytosis in adults: A case report and review of the literature. Medicine (Baltimore). 2016;**95**:e5431. DOI: 10.1097/MD.0000000000005431

[26] Amir AZ, Ling SC, Naqvi A, Weitzman S, Fecteau A, Grant D, et al. Liver transplantation for children with acute liver failure associated with secondary hemophagocytic lymphohistiocytosis. Liver Transplantation. 2016;**22**:1245-1253. DOI: 10.1002/lt.24485

[27] Guthery SL, Heubi JE. Liver involvement in childhood histiocytic syndromes. Current Opinion in Gastroenterology. 2001;**17**:474-478

[28] Capel MS, Hader I, Amin M. Acute liver failure secondary to severe systemic disease from fatal hemophagocytic lymphohistiocytosis: Case report and systematic literature review. World Journal of Hepatology. 2018;**10**:629-636. DOI: 10.4254/wjh.v10.i9.629

Chapter 8

Primary Sclerosing Cholangitis (PSC) in Children

Sabina Wiecek

Abstract

Primary sclerosing cholangitis (PSC) is a chronic liver disease of unknown aetiology affecting extrahepatic and/or intrahepatic bile ducts causing its inflammation and fibrosis with most frequent consequences including biliary cirrhosis and liver failure. The incidence of PSC in children and adolescents is 0.2 per 100,000 children per year, when in adults the reported incidence is higher and equals 0.5 to 1 in 100,000 individuals per year. PSC is more common among men and boys. The diagnosis is usually established in the second decade of life in the paediatric population with the mean age of diagnosis of 13.8 years. Many studies point out a strong correlation between IBD and PSC, especially ulcerative colitis. The prevalence of IBD among children with PSC diagnosis varies from 60 to 99%; however, the incidence of PSC is about 12% in patients with ulcerative colitis and fluctuates about 2–5% in Crohn's disease diagnosed patients. Clinical symptoms are present in approximately half of cases and they are unspecific in many of them. Elevated liver enzymes and biochemical markers of cholestasis are sometimes the only signs of PSC. Gold standard for PSC diagnosis is magnetic resonance cholangiopancreatography (MRCP) as a non-invasive procedure comparing to endoscopic retrograde cholangiopancreatography (ERCP) which is also used in some cases. The aim of the study was to review the risk factors, clinical symptoms, diagnostic methods and treatment of paediatric patients with primary sclerosing cholangitis.

Keywords: primary sclerosing cholangitis, children

Primary sclerosing cholangitis (PSC) is a chronic liver disease of unknown aetiology affecting extrahepatic and/or intrahepatic bile ducts causing its inflammation and fibrosis with most frequent consequences including biliary cirrhosis and liver failure. The incidence of PSC in children and adolescents is 0.2 per 100,000 children per year when in adults the reported incidence is higher and equals 0.5 to 1 in 100,000 individuals per year. Several studies indicate the incidence of primary sclerosing cholangitis is increasing. A similar increase has been seen in most autoimmune diseases. PSC is more common among men and boys. The diagnosis is usually established in the second decade of life in the paediatric population with the mean age of diagnosis of 13.8 years [1–9].

Many studies point out a strong correlation between IBD and PSC, especially ulcerative colitis. The prevalence of IBD among children with PSC diagnosis varies from 60 to 99%, however the incidence of PSC is about 12% in patients with ulcerative colitis and fluctuates about 2 to 5% in Crohn's disease diagnosed patients. In children, the diagnosis of IBD generally precedes the diagnosis of PSC [10–15].

1. Aetiology

The pathogenesis of PSC is unknown, but a number of mechanistic theories have been proposed. Despite the lack of scientifically proven aetiological factors, many components can be responsible for the PSC development.

1.1 Genetic background

Genetic background including an impact of HLA-A1, B8, DR3 haplotypes are one of the suspects as the diagnosis is made at a young age and family occurrence has been reported. Genome-wide comparisons of the frequency of genetic variants have provided a means of dissecting genetic risk in the many human diseases primary sclerosing cholangitis included. In the pathogenesis of PSC can play the role the presence of more non-HLA genes related to immunity and/or bile homeostasis. However most PSC genes appear to relate to adaptive immune reactions. There are limited genetic links between IBD and PSC. The HLA class 1 (expressed on all cells) and HLA class II (expressed on antigen- presenting cells) present potentially antigenic peptides derived from intra- and extracellular sources, to the T cell receptor (TCR) on CD* and CD4 T cells. But the antigenic peptides are unknown. Data suggest the presence of PSC specific TCR in the livers of patients. The predominant cell type in the portal inflammatory infiltrate in liver patients with primary sclerosing cholangitis is the T cell. It is suggested that there is cross-reaction between cholangiocytes and T-cells. Some of scientists believe that genes as PRDX5, TGR5, PSMG1, NFKB1 may play a role in innate immune reactions [11, 16–18].

1.2 Bile acids toxicity

The concentric fibrosis around the bile ducts in PSC is found in a variety of conditions and likely represents a final pathway for bile ducts injury. Defects of mechanisms protecting against bile acid toxicity can be a factor playing an important role in PSC development. The biliary epithelium shows an activated phenotype in PSC, including an expansion of the peribiliary gland system [19–21].

1.3 Autoimmunologic factors

What is more, certain autoimmune reactions in genetically susceptible individuals seem to play an important role as well. The presence of non-specific autoantibodies such as ANA, ANCA (in >80% of patients) and anti-SMA (in >60% of patients) together with autoimmune diseases such as autoimmune hepatitis (overlap syndrome PSC/AIH in 25–35%), rheumatoid arthritis, autoimmune thyroiditis or type 1 diabetes mellitus suggests that PSC can be described as an autoimmune disease. However its prevalence among men (2:1) and the lack of response to immunosuppressive therapy contributed to the concept of PSC being rather an immune-mediated disease. PSC with high immunoglobulin 4 (IgG4) levels and autoimmune hepatitis overlap syndrome have been described. But the lack of the efficacy of immunosuppressive treatment despite isolated autoimmune aetiology [11, 22–25].

1.4 Role of microbiota

The predominant coexistence of PSC and IBD led to a theory that dysregulation of gut microbiota in IBD patients causes liver T-cell activation provoking an inflammatory response in bile ducts. There is increasing appreciation of the co-metabolic functions of the gut microbiota in the bile homeostasis. The composition of the gut microbiota in PSC has been described using sequencing technologies. However, data from other diseases suggests that reduced bacterial diversity occurs prior to and independent from clinical manifestations [26–29].

2. Clinical picture

Clinical symptoms are present in approximately half of cases and they are unspecific in many of them. Most frequently patients complain of abdominal pain, fatigue and/or abdominal pain. Malaise, jaundice, splenomegaly or pruritus are reported less often. Elevated liver enzymes and biochemical markers of cholestasis are sometimes the only signs of PSC. The diagnosis of PSC may precede that of IBD, which may even present after liver transplantation for PSC. PSC may present in an IBD patients even after colectomy. Multiple gallbladder abnormalities in the course of primary sclerosing cholangitis including: dilatation (15%), gallstones (25%), cholecystitis, hydrops, polyps (4–6%), carcinoma (2.5–3.5%) are observed more often in patients [2, 8, 17, 22, 29, 30].

2.1 Forms of PSC

1. **Classical large-duct PSC**.

2. **Small-duct PSC**. A diagnosis of small-duct PSC is made upon histological findings characteristic of PSC and clinical and biochemical abnormalities suggestive of PSC. The HLA associations with IBD in small-duct PSC resemble those of large-duct PSC and suggest shared aetiologies between large-duct PSC and small -duct PSC in the presence of IBD.

3. **PSC with high IgG4**. PSC patients with elevated IgG4 are less responsive and data suggest they may progress more rapidly than other PSC patients. IgG4 may be involved in the pathogenesis of autoimmune cholangitis and clinical response upon treatment with the anti-CD20 antibody (rituximab).

4. **PSC-AIH overlap syndrome**. Biochemical and histological features of autoimmune hepatitis are apparent in 7–14% of patients with PSC. Elevated transaminases and IgG may indicate autoimmune hepatitis, but may be elevated as a part of the biliary disease.

5. **PSC with cholangiocarcinoma**.

3. Diagnostics

The diagnosis is based on laboratory and imaging results as well as on elimination of other than PSC cholestatic diseases. When it comes to laboratory results among children, gamma-glutamyltransferase (GGT) is more specific cholestatic marker than alkaline phosphatase (ALP) as ALP levels tend to fluctuate during bone growth. Even though ultrasound (USG) is a cheap and simple way to visualise liver pathology, bile ducts abnormalities characteristic of PSC might not be visible. Gold standard for PSC diagnosis is magnetic resonance cholangiopancreatography (MRCP) with acceptable sensitivity and specificity as a non-invasive procedure comparing to endoscopic retrograde cholangiopancreatography (ERCP) which is also used in some cases. As typical cholangiographic changes define the diagnosis of PSC, prognostic scoring system. To diagnose small duct PSC which is a type of PSC affecting intrahepatic ducts only, as well as to confirm the presence of PSC/AIH overlap syndrome it is necessary to perform liver histology. In recent years, there has been interest in the development of noninvasive tests of liver fibrosis for stratification and prognosis in PSC. Serum tests of liver fibrosis reflect fibrogenesis (APRI, Fib4 score). Liver stiffness measurement by transient elastography has been validated for the assessment of liver fibrosis in the liver diseases. Elastography in patients with PSC well correlate with the degree of fibrosis, performing best at the extremes of histological stage [5, 11, 31–34].

3.1 Differential diagnosis of PSC

1. Choledocholithiasis.
2. Congenital abnormalities of bile duct.
3. Cholangiocarcinoma without PSC.
4. Traumatic/ischemic changes in bile ducts.
5. HIV infection.
6. Infestation (ascaris, lambliosis)
7. Sarcoidosis.
8. Pyogenic cholangitis

3.2 Patients with PSC need control every 6 months

- Clinical review
- Serum liver tests
- Tumour marker: Ca 19-9, AFP
- Ultrasonography examination
- MRI/MRC if cirrhosis

4. Prognosis and complications

PSC is a progressive disease where bile ducts fibrosis lead to cirrhosis and liver failure. PSC has a highly variable natural history. Asymptomatic patients have been shown to have a better prognosis than patients with symptoms at diagnosis. Comparing to adults, PSC in children seems milder, yet 15–45% of paediatric patients will require liver transplantation within 6–12 years after the diagnosis. The increased risk of biliary cancer and colorectal cancer in PSC is firmly established and of major clinical importance. The risk of cholangiocarcinoma (CCA) is about 160 times higher than in the general population. In spite of that, only 1% of patients experience this serious complication. In a multi-centre study of 7000 PSC patients hepatobiliary malignancy was diagnosed in 10.9%. Up to 50% of cholangiocarcinoma are detected within a year of PSC diagnosis. Unfortunately, PSC diagnosed children may also develop other types of cancers such as gallbladder, colon or hepatocellular cancer. In the majority of cases, the early stages of cholangiocarcinoma are asymptomatic. Sometimes are observed abdominal pain, weight loss, increasing jaundice. Diagnosis of cholangiocarcinoma is based on tumour marker Ca19-9, imaging modalities, biliary brush cytology. The indication for liver transplantation in patients with dysplasia and no signs of cholangiocarcinoma remain controversial. Presence of dysplasia of any grade has been reported in 83% of explant livers with PSC-cholangiocarcinoma and 36% without cholangiocarcinoma. MRI and CT may visualise early features of cholangiocarcinoma in PSC but difficulties in distinguishing inflammatory, bening and malignant lesions lead to suboptimal diagnostic accuracy. Combined MRI/cholangioMRI has the highest sensitivity and specificity and is preferred for detection of small focus cholangiocarcinoma. Liver transplantation or surgery with complete resection is the only treatments with curative intent for cholangiocarcinoma. Liver transplantation with neoadjuvant therapy (external beam radiotherapy, endoluminal brachytherapy, chemotherapy) can be considered in patients with unresectable, perihilar early stage. Systemic chemotherapy remains the palliative treatment for patients not eligible for surgery. Other palliative treatment strategies include endoscopic stenting and photodynamic therapy.

PSC-IBD whether considered UC or Crohn's disease is almost universally colonic (usually a pancolitis) with a right-sided predominance, backwash ileitis and rectal sparing. The risk of colorectal cancer is fivefold higher than in IBD without PSC and may occur at any time from diagnosis. Colonoscopy should be performed in patients with PSC regularly from the moment of diagnosis. Chromoendoscopy is being increasingly recommended to facilitate detection of flat lesions with dysplasia. Four quadrant biopsies from all colonic segments and the terminal ileum should be performed. Hepatocellular and pancreatic cancer also occur in patients with PSC, but frequencies are lower than in cirrhosis liver from other causes. Currently there are no established prognostic tools that reliably estimate prognosis of the patients [2, 35–46].

5. Treatment

Effective ways of PSC treatment are still lacking. Immunosuppressive medications did not show any benefits, while oral vancomycin therapy might be an option although more data is required. Symptomatic treatment of PSC also consists of supplementing the deficiencies of fat-soluble vitamins, preventing the development of osteoporosis and combating chronic itching: by using additional cholestyramine at a dose of 6–8 g/24 h and/or rifampicin. For patients refractory to the above-mentioned treatment, oral naloxone therapy (50 mg/24 h) may be effective.

5.1 Ursodeoxycholic acid

Ursodeoxycholic acid (UDCA) is commonly used and has been proved to reduce GTP and AP levels which are both good prognostic factors improving patients' survival. However, UDCA treatment did not result in improved outcomes compared to no intervention. New therapeutic applications have been derived from this research in the form of norUDCA, to enhance general resistance to bile acid induced biliary injury. NorUDCA is slightly amidated in the liver, it is secreted into the bile in both unbound and glucuronic acid form. The biliary-hepatic flow of unbound norUDCA induces excessive secretion of bile rich in bicarbonate. Studies in mouse models have shown that the drug is less toxic, more effectively prevents peripheral fibrosis, proliferation of hepatocytes and cholangiocytes, reduces the content of hydroxyproline and infiltrating immune cells. In addition, it improves cholestasis parameters [6, 31, 47–48].

5.2 Vankomycin

Antibiotics, particularly vancomycin, may have a positive effect on PSC either via direct effects on the microbiome or via host-mediated mechanisms. In addition vancomycin has possible immunomodulatory and anti-inflammatory mechanisms, But there is not currently sufficient evidence to support treatment recommendations. Further research is needed to establish if vancomycin is a PSC treatment [48–50].

5.3 ERCP

Bile duct strictures are possible complications in the course of the disease that can be treated with prothesis during ERCP. The generally accepted arbitrary definition is stenosis of <1.5 mm in the common bile duct or <1 mmin the hepatic duct within 2 cm of the hilum. The incidence of complications associated with ERCP in patients with PSC is 4–18% [44, 46, 48].

5.4 Liver transplantation

Liver transplantation is a life-saving procedure with generally good outcomes, however, up to 16% of paediatric patients are affected by recurrent primary sclerosing cholangitis (rPSC) after transplantation. The indications for liver transplantation in PSC are similar to other liver diseases and transplanted with a qualifying MELD/PELD score in a patient with cirrhosis [11, 29, 51].

5.5 Treatment of bacterial cholangitis

Cholangitis occurs frequently but symptoms may be atypical. Prophylactic antibiotics should be ordered prior to and following biliary interventions. Positive bacterial or fungal cultures of bile can be associated with worse prognosis. Sometimes patients with recurrent cholangitis require long-term, rotating antibiotics.

Author details

Sabina Wiecek
Department of Paediatrics, Medical University of Silesia, Katowice, Poland

*Address all correspondence to: sabinawk@wp.pl

References

[1] Adike A, Carey EJ, Lindor KD. Primary sclerosing cholangitis in children versus adults: Lessons for the clinic. Expert Review of Gastroenterology & Hepatology. 2018;**12**:1025-1032

[2] Deneau M, Jensen MK, Holmen J, et al. Primary sclerosing cholangitis, autoimmune hepatitis, and overlap in Utah children: Epidemiology and natural history. Hepatology. 2013;**58**: 1392-1400

[3] Fagundes E, Ferreira A, Hosken C, et al. Primary sclerosing cholangitis in children and adolescent. Arquivos de Gastroenterologia. 2017;**54**:286-290

[4] Jankowska I. Pierwotne stwardniające zapalenie dróg żółciowych. In: Pediatria I, editor. Redakcja naukowa Wanda Kawalec, Ryszard Grenda, Marek Kulus. Warszawa: PZWL Wydawnictwo Lekarskie; 2018. p. 575

[5] Lindor KD, Kowdley KV, Harrison ME. American college of gastroenterology. ACG clinical guideline: Primary sclerosing cholangitis. The American Journal of Gastroenterology. 2015;**110**:646-659

[6] Mieli-Vergani G, Vergani D, Baumann U, et al. Diagnosis and management of paediatric autoimmune liver disease: ESPGHAN Hepatology committee position statement. Journal of Pediatric Gastroenterology and Nutrition. 2018;**66**:345-360

[7] Miloh T, Arnon R, Shneider B, et al. A retrospective single-center review of primary sclerosing cholangitis in children. Clinical Gastroenterology and Hepatology. 2009;**7**:239-245

[8] Weismuller T, Trivedy P, Bergquist A, et al. Patient age, sex and inflammatory bowel disease phenotypeassociate with course of primary sclerosing cholangitis. Gastroenterology. 2017;**152**:1975-1984

[9] Valentino PL, Wiggins S, Harney S, et al. The natural history of primary sclerosing cholangitis in children: A large single-center longitudinal cohort study. Journal of Pediatric Gastroenterology and Nutrition. 2016;**63**(6):603-609

[10] de Vries AB, Janse M, Blokzijl H, et al. Distinctive inflammatory bowel disease phenotype in primary sclerosing cholangitis. World Journal of Gastroenterology. 2015;**21**:1956-1971

[11] Karlsen T, Melum E, Franke A, et al. The utility of genome-wide association studies in hepatology. Hepatology. 2010;**51**:1833-1842

[12] Loftus EV Jr, Harewood GC, Loftus CG, et al. PSC-IBD: A unique form of inflammatory bowel disease associated with primary sclerosing cholangitis. Gut. 2005;**54**(1):91-96

[13] Mertz A, Nguyen NA, Katsanos KH, et al. Primary sclerosing cholangitis and inflammatory bowel disease comorbidity: An update of the evidence. Annals of Gastroenterology. 2019;**32**(2):124-133

[14] Naess S, Bjornsson E, Anmarkrud J, et al. Small-duct primary sclerosing cholangitis without inflammatory bowel disease is genetically different from large duct disese. Liver International. 2014;**34**:1488-1495

[15] Palmela C, Peerani F, Castaneda D, et al. Inflammatory bowel disease and primary sclerosing cholangitis: A review of the phenotype and associated specific features. Gut and Liver. 2018;**12**(1):17-29

[16] Karlsen TH, Folseraas T, Thorburn D, et al. Primary sclerosing cholangitis a comprehensive review. Journal of Hepatology. 2017;**67**(6):1298-1323

[17] Boberg K, Chapman R, Hirschfield G, et al. Overlap syndrome : The International Autoimmune Hepatitis Group (IAIHG) position statement on a controversial issue. Journal of Hepatology. 2011;**54**:374-385

[18] Pollheimer MJ, Halilbasic E, Fickert P, et al. Pathogenesis of primary sclerosing cholangitis. Best Practice & Research. Clinical Gastroenterology. 2011;**25**(6):727-739

[19] Alvaro D, Gigliozzi A, Artili A. Regulation and deregulation of cholangiocyte proliferation. Journal of Hepatology. 2000;**33**:333-340

[20] Bilhartz L. Gallstones Disease and its Complications. 6th ed. Saunders; 1998. p. 1-27

[21] Carpino C, Cardinale V, Renzi A, et al. Activation of biliary tree stem cells within peribiliary glands in primary sclerosing cholangitis. Journal of Hepatology. 2015;**63**:1220-1228

[22] Deneau MR, Mack C, Abdou R, et al. Gamma glutamyltransferase reduction is associated with favorable outcomes in pediatric primary sclerosing cholangitis. Hepatology Communications. 2018;**2**:1369-1378

[23] Maillette de Buy Wenniger L, Rauws E, Beuers U. What an endoscopist should know about immunoglobulin-G4-associated disease of the pancreas and biliary tree. Endoscopy. 2012;**44**:66-73

[24] Ponsioen C, Kuiper H, Ten K, et al. Immunohistochemical analysis of inflammation in primary sclerosing cholangitis. European Journal of Gastroenterology & Hepatology. 1999;**11**:769-774

[25] Whiteside T, Lasky S, Si L, et al. Immunologic analysis of mononuclear cells in liver tissues and blood of patients with primary sclerosing cholangitis. Hepatology. 1985;**5**:468-474

[26] Kevans D, Tyler A, Holm K, et al. Characterization of intestinal microbiota in ulcerative colitis patients with and without primary sclerosing cholangitis. Journal of Crohn's & Colitis. 2016;**10**:330-337

[27] Kummen M, Holm K, Anmarkrud J, et al. The gut microbial profile in patients with primary sclerosing cholangitis is distinct from patients with ulcerative colitis without biliary disease and healthy controls. Gut. 2017;**66**:611-619

[28] Quraishi M, Sergeant M, Kay G, et al. The gut-adherent microbiota of PSC–IBD is distinct to that of IBD. Gut. 2017;**66**:386-388

[29] Laborda TJ, Kyle Jense M, et al. Treatment of primary sclerosing cholangitis in children. World Journal of Hepatology. 2019;**11**(1):19-36

[30] Bjimsson E. Small-duct primary sclerosing cholangitis. Current Gastroenterology Reports. 2009;**11**:37-41

[31] Chapman R, Fevery J, Kalloo A, et al. Diagnosis and management of primary sclerosing cholangitis. Hepatology. 2010;**51**(2):660-678

[32] Corpechot C, Gaouar F, El Naggar A, et al. Baseline values and changes in the liver stiffness measured by transient elastogtaphy are associated with severity of fibrosis and outcome of patients with primary sclerosing cholangitis. Gastroenterology. 2014;**146**:970-979

[33] Deneau MR, El-Matary W, Valentino PL, et al. The natural history of primary sclerosing cholangitis in 781 children: A multicenter, international collaboration. Hepatology. 2017;**66**(2):518-527

[34] Ehlken H, Wroblewski R, Corpechot C, et al. Validation of

transient elastography and comparison with spleen length measurement for staging of fibrosis and clinical prognosis in primary sclerosing cholangitis. PLoS One. 2016;**11**:e0164224

[35] Blechacz B, Gores G. Cholangiocarcinoma: Advances in pathogenesis, diagnosis and treatment. Hepatology. 2008;**48**:308-321

[36] Boberg K, Ling G. Primary sclerosing cholangitis and malignancy. Best Practice & Research. Clinical Gastroenterology. 2011;**25**:753-764

[37] Broome U, Olsson R, Loof L, et al. Natural history and prognostic factors in 305 Swedish patients with with primary sclerosing cholangitis. Gut. 1996;**38**:610-615

[38] Burak K, Angulo P, Pasha TM, et al. Incidence and risk factors for cholangiocarcinoma in primary sclerosing cholangitis. The American Journal of Gastroenterology. 2004;**99**:523-526

[39] Charatcharoenwitthaya P, Enders F, Halling K, et al. Utility of serum tumor markers, imaging and biliary cytology for detecting cholangiocarcinoma in primary sclerosing cholangitis. Hepatology. 2008;**48**:1106-1117

[40] Feldstein AE, Perrault J, El-Youssif M, et al. Primary sclerosing cholangitis in children: A long-term follow-up study. Hepatology. 2003;**38**(1):210-217

[41] Kaminski M, Hassan C, Bisschops R, et al. Advanced imaging for detection and differentiation of colorectal neoplasia: European Society of Gastrointestinal Endoscopy (ESGE) Guideline. Endoscopy. 2014;**46**:435-449

[42] Levy C, Lymp J, Angulo P, et al. The value of serum Ca 19-9 in predicting of cholangiocarcinomas in patients with primary sclerosing cholangitis. Digestive Diseases and Sciences. 2005;**50**:1734-1740

[43] Nathan H, Pawlik T, Wolfgang C, et al. Trends in survivalafter surgery for cholangiocarcinoma: A 30 year population-based SEER database analysis. Journal of Gastrointestinal Surgery. 2007;**11**:1488-1496

[44] Rudolf G, Gotthardt D, Kloters-Plachky P, et al. Influence of dominant bile duct stenosis and biliary infections on outcome in primary sclerosing cholangitis. Journal of Hepatology. 2009;**51**:149-155

[45] Subramanian V, Mannath J, Ragunath K, et al. Meta-analysis: The diagnostic of chronoendoscopy for detecting dysplasia in patients with colonic inflammatory bowel disease. Alimentary Pharmacology & Therapeutics. 2011;**33**:304-312

[46] Stiehl A, Rudolf G, Kloters-Plachky P, et al. Development of dominant bile duct stenosis in patients with primary sclerosing cholangitis treated with ursodeoxycholic acid: Outcome after endoscopic treatment. Journal of Hepatology. 2002;**36**:151-156

[47] Lindor K, Kowdley R, Luketic V, et al. High-dose ursodeoxycholic acid for the treatment of primary sclerosing cholangitis. Hepatology. 2009;**50**:808-814

[48] Damman JL, Rodriguez EA, Ali AH, et al. Review article: The evidence that vancomycin is a therapeutic option for primary sclerosing cholangitis. Alimentary Pharmacology & Therapeutics. 2018;**47**:886-895

[49] Hey P, Lokan J, Johnson P, et al. Efficacy of oral vancomycin in recurrent primary sclerosing cholangitis following liver transplantation. BML Case Reports. 2017;**25**:2017. pii:bcr-2017-221165. DOI: 10.1136/bcr-2017-221165

[50] Shah A, Crawford D, Burger D, Martin N, et al. Effects of antibiotic therapy in primary sclerosing cholangitis with and without inflammatory bowel disease: A systematic review and meta-analysis. Seminars in Liver Disease. 2019;**39**(4):432-441

[51] Soufi N, Bazerbachi F, Deneau M. Post-transplant disease recurrence in pediatric PSC. Current Gastroenterology Reports. 2018;**20**:44. DOI: 10.1007/s11894-018-0649-2

Chapter 9

Cholestasis: The Close Relationship between Bile Acids and Coenzyme Q10

Manuela R. Martinefski, Silvia E. Lucangioli, Liliana G. Bianciotti and Valeria P. Tripodi

Abstract

Cholestasis is defined as the impairment in formation or excretion of bile from the liver to the intestine. It may result from defects in intrahepatic production of bile, impairment of hepatic transmembrane transporters, or mechanical obstruction to bile flow. In cholestasis, hepatocytes are exposed to high levels of bile acids, particularly those bearing hydrophobic properties. The increase in bile acids induces oxidative stress, leading to an imbalance in the prooxidant:antioxidant ratio which determines the final cellular redox status. This chapter will focus on the close relationship between bile acids and the most powerful endogenous antioxidant, coenzyme Q10 in cholestasis, and the eventual alternative therapeutic option of CoQ10 supplementation to current traditional therapies.

Keywords: cholestasis, coenzyme Q10, bile acids

1. Cholestasis: types, clinical presentation, diagnosis and current therapeutic approaches

Bile is a nonenzymatic secretion produced by hepatocytes. The main components of bile include bile salts necessary for enzymatic fat digestion and absorption, bilirubin, and cholesterol. Drugs and other xenobiotics are also excreted into bile following hepatic metabolization. Bile flow is dependent on the active canalicular transport of bile acids and other substrates mediated by the bile salt export pump (Bsep), which transports osmotically active monoanionic bile salts into the bile canaliculus and multidrug resistance-associated protein 2 (Mrp2), which exports oxidized and reduced glutathione. Bile secreted by the hepatocytes is stored and concentrated in the gallbladder, which contracts in the presence of the hormone cholecystokinin resulting in bile release into the duodenum through the cystic and common bile duct.

Cholestasis is defined as the decrease or suppression of bile flow due to impaired secretion by hepatocytes or to obstruction of bile at any level of the excretory pathway, from the hepatocyte canalicular membrane to the ampulla of Vater in the duodenum. Cholestasis leads to the retention of the major constituents of bile, bilirubin, and bile acids, in blood. By convention, cholestasis is chronic when it lasts more than 6 months. Prevalence of cholestasis is not significantly different between males and females. Nevertheless, women are at lighter risk of developing drug-induced cholestasis and intrahepatic cholestasis of pregnancy. Despite that, cholestasis may affect people of every age group, newborns and infants are more prone due to the immaturity of the liver.

The morphologic features of cholestasis are dependent on the severity, duration, and the underlying cause. Cholestasis is classified as intrahepatic or extrahepatic cholestasis depending on the cause that leads to impaired bile flow. Intrahepatic cholestasis is due to a disease affecting the hepatocytes and/or the intrahepatic bile ducts, whereas extrahepatic cholestasis or obstructive cholestasis results from the obstruction of the extrahepatic biliary ducts.

Obstruction of bile ducts can be caused by gallstones, cysts, stenosis, or tumors. The most frequent causes of extrahepatic cholestasis in adults include cholelithiasis and malignancies of the biliary tree or the head of the pancreas. However, in children, biliary atresia and cystic fibrosis are the main causes. Intermittent or partial obstruction may lead to ascending cholangitis, a secondary bacterial infection of the biliary tree. The typical morphological changes are reversible if the obstruction is corrected, but if it persists it can lead to biliary cirrhosis.

Causes of intrahepatic or hepatocellular cholestasis include viral and autoimmune hepatitis, inborn errors of bile acid synthesis, primary biliary cirrhosis, progressive familial intrahepatic cholestasis, primary sclerosing cholangitis, total parenteral nutrition, and drug toxicity. The drug class mostly implicated in cholestasis is antibiotics. However, anti-inflammatory drugs, highly active antiretroviral therapy, psychotropes, some chemotherapy agents, oral contraceptives, and anabolic steroids have also been reported to cause cholestasis [1]. Although primary sclerosing cholangitis affects intrahepatic bile ducts, it can also affect extrahepatic bile ducts.

Clinical presentation of cholestasis includes jaundice, pruritus, skin xanthomas, or symptoms associated with intestinal malabsorption. Jaundice and pruritus are present in all types of cholestasis whether acute or chronic, whereas the other clinical features are more associated with chronic cholestasis.

Jaundice is the clinical expression of bilirubin retention. Excretion of conjugated bilirubin is the rate-limiting step of bilirubin clearance. During cholestasis, conjugation of bilirubin continues but the excretion is significantly reduced. Jaundice is observed by scleral icterus at a concentration as low as 2 mg/dL accompanied by dark urine. The concentration of conjugated bilirubin in blood depends on its production rate and excretion pathways, as well as cholestasis degree. Non conjugated bilirubin is also increased in patients with cholestasis. The magnitude of the increase in serum bilirubin concentration does not correlated with the type or severity of cholestasis. Pruritus is a frequent clinical manifestation of cholestasis, which has been long associated with increased serum bile acids. However, its origin is multifactorial and diverse studies show that not only bile acids but also lysophosphatidic acid, and bilirubin are potential mediators of cholestatic itch [2]. Retention of bile acids and their conjugated salts results in biological membrane injury, particularly in the liver due to their detergent properties. Increased hydrophobic bile salts favor their incorporation into membranes, altering membrane fluidity and function. Enhanced secondary bile acids like lithocholic acid result in further membrane injury. The transport of bile salts from plasma to bile is the principal driving force for bile formation and it is mediated by several hepatic transporters, mostly belonging to the ABC family of transporters. Numerous studies support that the failure to excrete bile salts into the canaliculus is the main mechanism underlying cholestasis. In this sense retrieval of the canalicular transporters Bsep and Mrp2 from hepatocyte plasma membrane to endosomal compartments in different types of cholestasis has been well documented [3, 4]. However, other works consider that the endocytic retrieval of canalicular transporter is the result of cholestasis on the hepatocyte function. In either case, the retention of bile salts in the liver induces down-regulation of bile acid synthesis, overall reduction in the total pool size and damage to hepatocytes.

Skin xanthomas and signs of malabsorption are associated with chronic cholestasis. Skin xanthomas result from focal accumulation of cholesterol in the dermis and usually appear around the eyes, but may be present in other parts of the body. Malabsorption occurs due to the failure of enough bile salts to reach the duodenum, so the digestion and absorption of dietary fat is impaired. Fat soluble vitamins like A, E, D, and K are poorly absorbed in cholestasis leading to clinical symptoms and signs of their deficiency.

In all types of cholestasis, characteristic laboratory findings are elevated serum alkaline phosphatase and γ-glutamyltranspeptidase, enzymes present on the canalicular membranes of hepatocytes, and bile duct epithelial cells. Alkaline phosphatase is also elevated in bone growth or disease, pregnancy, or intestinal diseases. λ-Glutamyltranspeptidase is a sensitive marker of cholestasis [5], although no specific since it can be elevated in other liver diseases [6]. Furthermore, its elevation may reflect enzyme induction by drugs or alcohol. Serum 5′-nucleotidase, an enzyme located in canalicular membranes and lining the sinusoids is also elevated in cholestasis, although it appears to be less sensitive than alkaline phosphatase. Serum elevation of hepatic enzymes is accompanied by increased serum bilirubin and bile acids. An increase in serum bile acids is an early marker of cholestasis.

In the diagnosis of cholestasis, the first key step is to identify whether it is intrahepatic, extrahepatic, or both. The patient history and physical examination usually provide useful information. Elevation of both hepatic enzymes (alkaline phosphatase and λ-glutamyl transpeptidase) is a hallmark of cholestasis although the identification of the type of cholestasis requires imaging studies and additional biochemical studies. Imaging studies include first an abdominal ultrasonography to exclude dilated intra and extrahepatic ducts. When bile duct alterations are observed, further imaging studies like magnetic resonance cholangiopancreatography or endoscopic retrograde cholangiopancreatography should be performed. A diagnostic of intrahepatic cholestasis can be made when imaging studies exclude mechanical obstruction. Then, further biochemical studies are necessary to identify the intrahepatic cause of cholestasis, including liver biopsies when the diagnosis is unclear.

The therapeutic intervention for cholestasis may differ depending on the etiology [7]. Based on controlled clinical trials, ursodeoxycholic acid (UDCA) is the treatment of choice for diverse cholestatic disorders like primary biliary cirrhosis and intrahepatic cholestasis of pregnancy due to its anticholestatic properties. However, UDCA treatment is not so effective in other cholestatic disorders like in primary sclerosing cholangitis. No therapy of proven benefit for the long-term prognosis of genetic cholestatic liver disease exists. In drug-induced cholestasis, withdrawal of the drug is the only effective treatment [8]. Pruritus is a common manifestation of cholestasis, which can be of serious severity. Management of pruritus includes cholestyramine as first line-treatment and then rifampicin, and opiate antagonists [9].

2. Bile acids: physicochemical properties, synthesis, and therapeutics

2.1 Bile acids physicochemical properties

Bile acids (BA) are steroid compounds, hydroxyl derivatives of 5β-cholan-24 oic acid. Primary BA are cholic acid (CA) and chenodeoxycholic acid (CDCA);

secondary BA such as deoxycholic acid (DCA) and lithocholic acid (LCA), all of them in 3α-position, and ursodeoxycholic acid (UDCA) is a hydroxyl derivative in 3β-position (**Figure 1**) [10].

BA have different physicochemical properties according to the number, position, and orientation of their hydroxy groups and the conjugation with glycine and taurine (**Figure 1**). In this sense, this characteristic influence their solubility, detergency, and hydrophobicity [11].

BA have an important role in biological systems under physiological and pathological conditions [12]. Their functions are associated with lipid digestion and absorption, solubilization of cholesterol and bile formation. In this case, BA influence in volume and composition of the bile.

The number, position, and orientation of the hydroxy groups of the BA impact directly on the hydrophobicity and detergency property and the relationship to the toxicity. In the case of BA with hydroxy groups in 3-α position, the higher the number of hydroxy groups, less hydrophobicity and lower detergency and, as a result, lower toxicity.

It must be pointed out that the orientation of the hydroxy group rules over the properties in the molecule. This can be seen on the CDCA (7α) and its epimer, the UDCA (7β), where the UDCA showed a strong reduction of detergency and hydrophobicity. Also, the BA toxicity is directly related to its hydrophobicity and detergency, because those interact with the cellular membranes in different ways, including the union, the insertion in the lipidic bilayer and its solubilization increasing its fluidity [10].

Therefore, UDCA is administered as therapeutic agent for the treatment of hepatobiliary disorders such as cholestasis, biliary dyspepsia, primary biliary cirrhosis, and different cholestatic conditions.

2.2 Bile acids synthesis

The synthesis of BA is produced exclusively in the liver, based on a series of enzymatic reactions in the hepatocyte, in which 17 enzymes are involved. The cholesterol (hydrophobic compound) turns into the primary BA, also known as colic acid (CA) and chenodeoxycholic (CDCA), through the first step and limiting of the called "classic" or "neutral" way of the BA biosynthesis, where the hydroxylation of the cholesterol is produced, catalyzed by the enzyme cytochrome P450

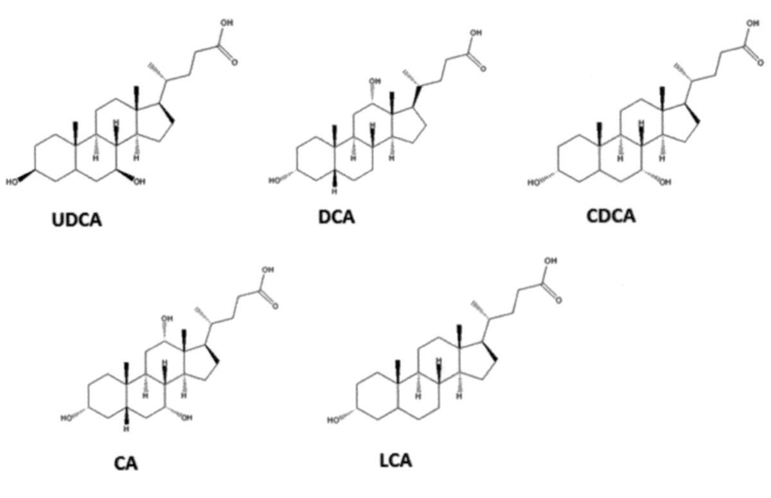

Figure 1.
Bile acids: chemical structure.

cholesterol 7a-hydroxylasa (CYP7A1). The BA synthesis can also occur through an "alternative" or "acidic" way, where the CYP27A1 intervenes and changes the BA oxysterols. Unlike the CYP7A1, the CYP27A1 is not regulated by the BA and is estimated only the 6% of the synthesis of BA is produced through this way. Before its secretion in the canalicular biliary light for the storage in the biliary gold bladder as mixed micelles with phospholipids and cholesterol, the primary BA are mainly conjugated with taurine and glycine, forming the conjugated BA, that with the Na^+ and K^+ form the biliary salts. When ingesting a food, the contraction of biliary gold bladder expels the micellar BA to the intestinal light to help digestion. In the gut, the intestinal bacteria deconjugate and dehydroxylate the primary BA, resulting in other species, denominated secondary BA: deoxycholic acid (DCA), a CA derivative, and ursodeoxycholic acid (UDCA), a CDCA derivative. The enterohepatic circulation allows the 95% of the BA to be reabsorbed from the distal ileum and transported back to the liver through portal circulation. Only 5% of the BA are not reabsorbed and are eliminated through feces. This small amount of loss is recovered through the novo synthesis of the BA in the liver. The size of the BA reserve is strictly regulated by the liver and gut to avoid a cytotoxic accumulation. When the reserve of BA increases, a feedback mechanism is activated, ruled by the interaction of several nuclear receptors, mainly the farnesoid X nuclear receptor (FXR) to inhibit the novo synthesis of BA. Therefore, the FXR is a "BA sensor," when the BA are joined to this receptor, they mediate their own synthesis control to provide a strict regulation of its reserve [13–15].

2.3 Bile acid therapy in hepatobiliary disease: role of UDCA

BA as therapeutic agent are appropriated in the chronic cholestasis deceases. BA can be orally administered following two strategies, the "displacement therapy" and/or "replacement therapy." UDCA may be used to displace endogenous BA to decrease the intrahepatic concentration of potentially cytotoxic BA accumulated in cholestasis. On the other hand, primary BA such as cholic acid (CA) might be used to replace a depleted BA pool resulted from defective biosynthesis on consequence to restore the physiological function of BA [16, 17].

UDCA (3α-7β-hydroxy-5β-cholan-24-oic acid) is naturally occurring BA, that normally constitutes 1–2% of the BA in human bile. UDCA is obtained by 7α-epimerization of the primary BA chenodeoxycholic acid (CDCA), by intestinal bacteria. [18] UDCA and CDCA differ in the hydroxyl group orientation at seventh position, allowing higher hydrophilicity of UDCA in comparison to CDCA.

UDCA is a weak acid (pKa = 5), and poorly water soluble, however, its solubility increases directly to the increase of the solution pH. After orally administrations, UDCA must be solubilized in mixed micelles present in small intestinal content in order to allow absorption [19, 20]. During the cholestasis disease, the UDCA bioavailability is limited due to the reduction of endogenous BA micelles in the duodenal lumen. Unconjugated UDCA is absorbed by passive diffusion in the proximal jejunum and in the ileum, thus extracted from portal venous blood by the liver and conjugated with glycine or taurine. Conjugated UDCA is secreted into the bile.

It is worth mentioning that in the UDCA oral administration, the half-life of the UDCA in the portal circulation is short, thus the maximum concentrations in liver/bile achieved by dividing the dose equally over 24 h are adequate.

UDCA is the BA of choice in view of the proven efficacy and lack of side effects in the treatment of cholestasis diseases. In the case of CDCA, its inherent toxicity is related to the fact that CDCA undergoes bacterial conversion dihydroxylation to a toxic, monohydroxy BA, like lithocholic acid (LCA), unlike UDCA, which is more resistant to bacterial dihydroxylation [21, 22].

The versatility presented by UDCA in the treatment of cholestatic diseases is due to its multiple action mechanisms:

- Biliary stones dilution
- Changes in the BA reserve hydrophobicity level
- Protection against the cellular death induced by cytotoxic BA
- Modulation of the expression of the transporters and the liver's enzymatic systems
- Normalization of the altered cellular location of hepatocellular transporters
- Immunoregulatory effects

2.3.1 Biliary stones dissolution

UDCA reduces the content of cholesterol in the bile by reducing the hepatic synthesis of cholesterol and its absorption by the gut itself. In addition to solubilizing the cholesterol into micelles, it causes the cholesterol to scatter into liquid crystals in an aqueous medium causing a favorable environment for the dissolution of biliary stones. In addition to this, reduces the viscosity and improves the bile flow.

2.3.2 Changes in the BA reserve levels of hydrophobicity

In the cholestasis, the increase of hydrophobic BA produces the cytolysis of plasmatic membrane. In normal individuals, the UDCA represents not more than 4% of the complete endogenous BA reserve. Under a treatment with UDCA, this percentage increases to 40–60% under a conventional dosage of 13–15 mg/kg/day, becoming the UDCA the predominant BA, which shifts the more hydrophobic endogenous BA. Therefore, the substitution of the potentially toxic hydrophobic endogenous BA in the total BA group to a hydrophilic turns the bile more hydrophilic and less cytotoxic, reducing the hepatic lesion.

2.4 UDCA and oxidative stress

It has been proposed that UDCA antioxidative action is due to the induction of glutathione (GSH) synthesis and in this way, mitochondrial injury apoptosis is prevented [23]. UDCA activates the phosphatidylinositol 3-kinase (PI3K)/Akt signaling pathway and induces the translocation of nuclear factor-E2-related factor 2 (Nrf2) into the nucleus. Hence, it could be hypothesized that UDCA increases the gene expression of enzymes associated with GSH synthesis and induces the down-regulation of intracellular ROS levels [24]. In a similar fashion, insulin reduces oxidative stress by the activation of PI3K and extracellular signal-regulated protein kinase in HepG2 cells [25]. Therefore, both UDCA and insulin may exert a cytoprotective effects against oxidative stress and. Noteworthy, UDCA may reduce fatty acids-induced insulin resistance.

3. Coenzyme Q10: generalities, clinical approaches and its relation to intrahepatic cholestasis of pregnancy

Coenzyme Q (CoQ) is an endogenous lipophilic compound synthetized in all tissues and cells. The biosynthetic pathway of CoQ in eukaryotes has been characterized by studies of mutants deficient in CoQ in *Saccharomyces cerevisiae*. The biosynthesis of CoQ initiates with the hydroxybenzoic acid to which a polyisoprenoid lipid tail is attached. Thus, CoQ is the product of two different converging biosynthetic pathways: the synthesis of 4-hydroxybenzoate, derived from the metabolism of tyrosine and the synthesis of the isoprene side chain that begins with the conversion of acetyl-coenzyme A (CoA) through the mevalonate route and regulated by the HMG CoA reductase. Formerly, the trans-prenyl transferase catalyzes the condensation of farnesyl pyrophosphate with numerous trans isopentenyl pyrophosphates, to form the long isoprenoid chain. Finally, these two pathways converge in a terminal step, where 4-hydroxybenzoate and polyprenyl pyrophosphate are linked by a condensation reaction catalyzed by the enzyme polyprenyl 4-hydroxybenzoate transferase [26].

Due to its ubiquitous distribution, CoQ is also called ubiquinone. In mammals, ubiquinone contains a 2,3-dimethoxy-5-methylbenzoquinone core with, predominantly, a hydrophobic 10 isoprenyl units, so it is designated as coenzyme Q10 (CoQ10, **Figure 2**).

CoQ10, mainly placed in the inner mitochondrial membrane, plays its principal role in promoting the electron transfer from complexes I and II to complex III within the mitochondrial respiratory chain to finally obtain cellular energy [27]. Taking into account its redox properties, CoQ10 also acts as a potent lipophilic antioxidant, scavenging oxygen reactive species, protecting lipids, protein, and cellular DNA and being involved in multiple steps of vital cellular metabolism such as the electron transfer in plasmatic membranes [28] and lysosomes [29], modulation of apoptosis [30, 31] and proton transport between uncoupled proteins [32]. CoQ10 also has an important intracellular signaling role in modulating the mitochondrial permeability transition pore [33].

Although its biosynthesis is not completely dilucidated, it is well known that different mutations in some genes which codify for proteins within its biosynthetic pathway have been identified. These mutations define the primary CoQ10 deficiencies [34–40]. At this time, from the 13 known CoQ genes direct or indirect related to CoQ biosynthesis, it is recognize that eight of them can cause CoQ10 deficiency and disease [41]. Primary CoQ10 deficiencies are a group of rare diseases of clinically heterogeneous appearance suggesting an autosomal recessive inheritance, because relatives are often affected, whereas parents are characteristically unaffected. The four most frequent clinical phenotypes associated with primary CoQ10 deficiencies are encephalomiophaty, cerebellar ataxia, multisystemic infantile form, and glomerulophaty and myophaty, all of them having a muscular and neurologic compromise [27]. Patients affected with primary CoQ10 deficiency, although its clinical severity, highly respond to CoQ10 supplementation being most effective the sooner the treatment begins [35, 42].

On the contrary, secondary CoQ10 deficiency is more frequent and of less severe clinical presentation. However, its treatment only ameliorates the symptoms although improve life quality. Secondary CoQ10 deficiency is associated to different pathologies such as neuro-muscular degenerative pathologies, cardiovascular, thyroid

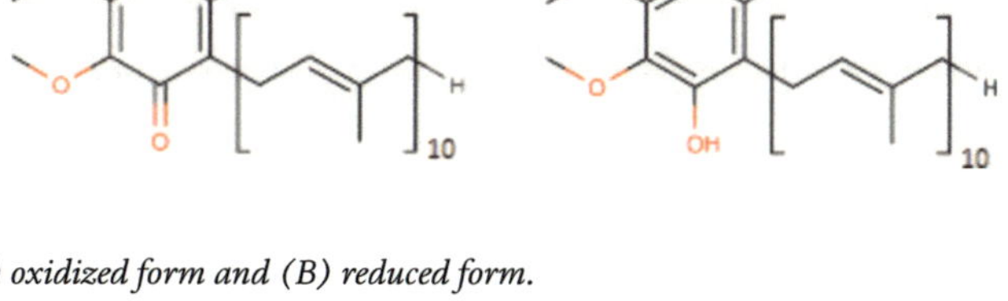

Figure 2.
Coenzyme Q10: (A) oxidized form and (B) reduced form.

and reproductive diseases as well as cancer among others [43–46]. Coenzyme Q10 deficiency is commonly found associated to mitochondrial oxidative phosphorylation impairment, probably as an adaptive mechanism to maintain a balance in mitochondrial redox status. However, in spite of the high incidence of secondary CoQ deficiencies, the precise mechanisms underlying these secondary deficiencies remain unidentified specially in non-mitochondrial oxidative phosphorylation disorders [47].

What is certain is that final cellular CoQ10 concentration is related to the balance existing between biosynthetic and dietary supply on one side and energetic consumption on the other [48].

In a previous work, we have demonstrated a reduced plasmatic level of CoQ10 in mothers with intrahepatic cholestasis of pregnancy (ICP) as well as in an animal model, being the first report connecting CoQ10 deficiency to this disorder [49]. Later, it was confirmed in another study, which analyzed fetal CoQ10 levels in cord blood from ICP mothers [50]. It is well known that ICP is a high-risk pregnancy disease characterized by the accumulation of total serum bile acids, with an enhanced proportion of the hydrophobic bile acids which are highly cytotoxic. During the last decade, it was found many evidences suggesting that hydrophobic bile acids increase is responsible for the higher oxidative stress observed in ICP [51–53]. Thus, it was reasonable to suspect that CoQ10 levels could be diminished, secondary to the oxidative stress and/or mediated by a metabolic feedback [50]. Furthermore, a depleted CoQ9 levels (the predominant form of ubiquinone in rodents) was also observed in plasma, brain and muscle in a cholestatic rat model together with a positive correlation between CoQ9 and ursodeoxycholic/lithocholic acid ratio (UDCA/LCA). The latter suggests that increased plasma LCA may be closely related to CoQ9 decrease in blood and tissues [49].

CoQ10 decrease in ICP possibly reveals a disturbance on the delicate balance between oxidative stress and antioxidant defenses, thus accumulating large amounts of free radicals, imparing energy production, and increasing risk for the fetus. Although the relationship between CoQ10 and serum bile acids is not well established, it is possible that reduced CoQ10 levels result from enhanced ubiquinone extraction from blood because of higher cellular demand. As it was previously mentioned, it is also probable that CoQ10 depletion may be caused by increased proportion of circulating and intracellular hydrophobic bile acids and enhanced consumption of the CoQ10 by free radicals and/or a metabolic down regulation. The relationship between CoQ and bile acids will be discussed in the next section.

Since CoQ10 is a potent antioxidant and is even proposed as the first line of defense against oxidative insult [54], its tissue distribution and plasma levels will be dependent on its susceptibility to the oxidative stress induced by cholestasis.

4. Bile acids and coenzyme Q10: possible relationship

Several studies have provided evidence that oxidative stress may play an important role in the pathogenesis of hepatic injury in animal models of cholestasis [52, 55–58] and in humans [59–61].

Hepatic mitochondria have been proposed as the most important cellular source of reactive oxygen species (ROS) induced by bile acids (BA). Hydrophobic BA impair respiration and electron transport in hepatic mitochondria. Krähenbühl et al. reported that hydrophobic BA decrease the activities of several enzyme complexes involved in the electron transport chain, such as complexes I, III, and IV but not affected complex II in isolated rat liver mitochondria. Furthermore, hydrophobic BA decrease the mitochondrial membrane potential developed upon succinate energization and decrease state three and enhance state four in mitochondria [62].

Yerushalmi et al. [63] proposed that ROS are generated at the ubiquinone-complex III interaction of the respiratory chain in hepatic mitochondria upon exposure to BA. Additionally, Botla et al. [64] reported that hydrophobic BA initiates the membrane permeability transition in hepatic mitochondria. In this context, oxidative stress results from an imbalance between increased free radical and impairment of antioxidant systems.

Therefore, the link between BA and CoQ has recently achieved clinical relevance and open to potential therapeutics challenges. As it was aforementioned, a study with a validated animal model of ICP, which shows similar biochemical hepatic alterations as observed in ICP patients, showed a significant decrease in CoQ9 and α-tocopherol in plasma that correlated negatively with the increase in LCA levels in the animal model of ICP [49]. Stocker and Bowry reported that CoQ acts earlier than α-tocopherol in the antioxidant system, thus the reduction of plasmic CoQ could be considered as an early marker of oxidative insult [54]. The decrease in these antioxidants may contribute to increase oxidative stress in ICP [49]. CoQ plasmatic levels more likely reflect the degree of metabolic request; in this case decreased levels may be related to consumption by free radicals or by increasing cellular demand. On the other hand, tissue CoQ levels are related to the balance between biosynthesis, dietary supply and energetic consumption [48]. The increase in BA has different effect over CoQ tissue levels. It was observed that skeletal muscle and brain were more susceptible to oxidative stress and showed a decrease in CoQ levels in ICP animals, whereas liver and heart content of CoQ remained unchanged. An hepatic paradox described in animal model of cholestasis including EE cholestasis, where the activity of HMG-CoA reductase and 7 alpha hydroxylase is increased despite the increase of BA, could possible explain this finding [65–68]. Thus, taking into account, that CoQ is synthesized via HMG-CoA reductase, it is possible that levels were maintained by an increase in its synthesis [49].

In accordance with those results, a significant decrease in CoQ10 and vitamin E levels was also observed in ICP patients respect to control pregnancies, coupled to an increase in total serum BA with a more hydrophobic profile [49]. It is worth mentioning that neonates are highly susceptible to oxidative damage caused by ROS, since the extrauterine environment is richer in oxygen than the intrauterine environment [69]. This problem is further aggravated by the low efficiency of natural antioxidant systems in the neonate that could be worsened if the antioxidant capacity of mother is deficient [48]. In addition, the direction of placental BA gradient, in normal pregnancy occurs from the fetus to the mother in order to promote toxic compounds elimination from the fetal compartment, while in ICP, this gradient is inverted allowing to accumulate BA in the fetal compartment [70, 71]. Thus, decreased CoQ10 levels in mothers with ICP may pose a risk for the newborn.

Recently, another study which evaluates umbilical cord blood of newborn from ICP mothers showed a decrease in cholesterol normalized CoQ10 content and an increase in total serum BA respect to normal pregnancy [50]. The results obtained by Martinefski et al. demonstrated a highly prooxidant environment.

Nowadays, since the relationship between CoQ and BA is not well established, two explanations have been hypothesized. On one hand, during ICP, cholesterol levels could possibly be maintained due to a mevalonate pathway deviation flow that absorbs another branch of the metabolic flow including those required to support CoQ synthesis [72].

On the other hand, hydrophobic BA stimulate the generation of ROS leading to a consumption of different antioxidants, including CoQ. Both scenarios led to a secondary CoQ deficiency.

In the field of cholestasis therapeutics, CoQ10 synthetic analog (idebenone) has shown to prevent BA stimulation of ROS from hepatic mitochondria and isolated hepatocytes [63]. Therefore, taking into account the deficiency of CoQ found in ICP, supplementation with CoQ10 could represent a new complementary therapeutic proposal for ICP in order to protect both the mother and the newborn. However, further studies are required to obtain a deeper conclusion.

Author details

Manuela R. Martinefski, Silvia E. Lucangioli, Liliana G. Bianciotti and Valeria P. Tripodi*
Facultad de Farmacia y Bioquimica, Universidad de Buenos Aires, Argentina

*Address all correspondence to: vtripodi@ffyb.uba.ar

References

[1] Fernández-Murga LM, Petrov PD, Conde I, Castell JV, Goméz-Lechón MJ, Jover R. Advances in drug-induced cholestasis: Clinical perspectives, potential mechanisms and in vitro systems. Food and Chemical Toxicology. 2018;**120**:196-212

[2] Patel SP, Vasavda C, Ho B, Meixiong J, Dong X, Kwatra SG. Cholestatic pruritus: Emerging mechanisms and therapeutics. Journal of the American Academy of Dermatology. 2019

[3] Miszczuk GS, Barosso IR, Larocca MC, Marrone J, Marinelli RA, Boaglio AC, et al. Mechanisms of canalicular transporter endocytosis in the cholestatic rat liver. Biochimica et Biophysica Acta - Molecular Basis of Disease. 2018;**1864**:1072-1085

[4] Roma MG, Barosso IR, Miszczuk G, Crocenzi FA, Pozzi EJS. Dynamic localization of hepatocellular transporters: Role in biliary excretion and impairment in cholestasis. Current Medicinal Chemistry. 2019;**26**:1113-1154

[5] Ozer J, Ratner M, Shaw M, Bailey W, Schomaker S. The current state of serum biomarkers of hepatotoxicity. Toxicology. 2008;**245**:194-205

[6] Giannini EG, Testa R, Savarino V. Liver enzyme alteration: A guide for clinicians. CMAJ. 2005;**72**:367-379

[7] EASL. European Association for the Study of the liver EASL clinical practice guidelines: Management of cholestatic liver diseases. Journal of Hepatology. 2009:237-267

[8] Navarro VJ, Senior JR. Drug-related hepatotoxicity. The New England Journal of Medicine. 2006;**354**:731-739

[9] Düll MM, Kremer AE. Treatment of pruritus secondary to liver disease. Current Gastroenterology Reports. 2019;**21**(9):48

[10] Roda A, Gioacchini AM, Manetta AC, Cerrè C, Montagnani M, Fini A. Bile acids: Physico-chemical properties, function and activity. Journal of Gastroenterology. 1995;**27**:327-331

[11] Lucangioli S, Carducci C, Tripodi V, Kenndler E. Retention of bile salts in micellar electrokinetic chromatography: Relation of capacity factor to octanol–water partition coefficient and critical micellar concentration. Journal of Chromatography B. 2001;**765**:113-120

[12] Hoffman A, Roda A. Physicochemical properties of bile acids and their relationshiio to biological properties: An overview of the problem. Journal of Lipid Research. 1984;**25**:1477-1488

[13] Stales B, Fonseca V. Bile acids and metabolic regulation: Mechanisms and clinical responses to bile acid sequestration. Diabetes Care. 2009;**32**(2):S237-S245

[14] Tonin F, Arends IWCE. Latest development in the synthesis of ursodeoxycholic acid (UDCA): A critical review. Beilstein Journal of Organic Chemistry. 2018;**14**:470-483

[15] Tripodi V, Lucangioli S, Scioscia S, Carducci C. Simultaneous determination of free and conjugated bile acids in serum by cyclodextrin-modified micellar electrokinetic chromatography. Journal of Chromatography B. 2003;**785**:147-155

[16] Balistreri W. Fetal and neonatal bile aids synthesis and metabolism-clinical implications. Journal of Inherited Metabolic Disease. 1991;**14**:459-477

[17] Hofmann A. Targeting drugs to the enterohepatic circulation: Lessons from bile acids and other endobiotics. Journal of Controlled Release. 1985;**2**:3-11

[18] Hofmann A. Pharmacology of ursodeoxycholic acid, and enterohepatic drug. Scandinavian Journal of Gastroenterology. 1994;**29**:S1-S15

[19] Aldini R, Montiagnani M, Roda A, Hrelia S, Biagi P, Roda E. Intestinal absorption of bile acid in the rabbit: Different transport rates in jejunum and ileum. Gastroenterology. 1996;**110**:458-459

[20] Bouscarel B, Nussbaum R, Dubner H, Fromm H. The roll of sodium in uptake of ursodeoxycholic acid in isolated hamster hepatocytes. Hepatology. 1995;**21**:145-154

[21] Cohen B, Hofmann A, Mosbach E. Differing effects of nor-ursodeoxycholic or ursodeoxycholic acid on hepatic histology and bile acid metabolism in the rabbit. Gastroenterology. 1986;**91**:189-197

[22] Palmer R. Bile acid, liver injury, and liver disease. Archives of Internal Medicine. 1972;**130**:606-617

[23] Mitsuyoshi H, Nakashima T, Sumida Y, Yoh T, Nakajima Y, Ishikawa H, et al. Ursodeoxycholic acid protects hepatocytes against oxidative injury via induction of antioxidants. Biochemical and Biophysical Research Communications. 1999;**263**:537-542

[24] Arisawa S, Ishida K, Kameyama N, Ueyama J, Hattori A, Tatsumi Y, et al. Ursodeoxycholic acid induces glutathione synthesis through activation of PI3K/Akt pathway in HepG2 cells. Biochemical Pharmacology. 2009;**77**:858-866

[25] Kang S, Song J, Kang H, Kim S, Lee Y, Park D. Insulin can block apoptosis by decreasing oxidative stress via phosphatidylinositol 3-kinase- and extracellular signal-regulated protein kinase-dependent signaling pathways in HepG2 cells. European Journal of Endocrinology. 2003;**148**:147-155

[26] Turunen M, Olsson J, Dallner G. Metabolism and function of coenzyme Q. Biochimica et Biophysica Acta. 2004;**1660**(1-2):171-199

[27] Quinzii C, Hirano M. Coenzyme Q and mitochondrial disease. Developmental Disabilities Research Reviews. 2010;**16**(2):183-188

[28] Sun IL, Sun EE, Crane FL, Morré DJ, Lindgren A, Löw H. Requirement for coenzyme Q in plasma membrane electron transport. Proceedings of the National Academy of Sciences of the United States of America. 1992;**89**:11126-11130

[29] Gille L, Nohl H. The existence of a lysosomal redox chain and the role of ubiquinone. Archives of Biochemistry and Biophysics. 2000;**375**:347-354

[30] Fontaine E, Ichas F, Bernardi P. A ubiquinone-binding site regulates the mitochondrial permeability transition pore. The Journal of Biological Chemistry. 1998;**273**:25734-25740

[31] Walter L, Miyoshi H, Leverve X, Bernard P, Fontaine E. Regulation of the mitochondrial permeability transition pore by ubiquinone analogs. A progress report. Free Radical Research. 2002;**36**:405-412

[32] Echtay KS, Winkler E, Klingenberg M. Coenzyme Q is an obligatory cofactor for uncoupling protein function. Nature. 2000;**408**:609-613

[33] Parikh S, Saneto R, Falk MJ, Anselm I, Cohen BH, Haas R. The mitochondrial medicine society. A modern approach to the treatment of mitochondrial disease. Current Treatment Options in Neurology. 2009;**11**(6):414-430

[34] Diomedi-Camassei F, Di Giandomenico S, Santorelli FM, Caridi G, Piemonte F, Montini G, et al.

COQ2 nephropathy: A newly described inherited mitochondriopathy with primary renal involvement. Journal of the American Society of Nephrology. 2007;**18**:2773-2780

[35] Duncan AJ, Bitner-Glindzicz M, Meunier B, Costello H, Hargreaves IP, López LC, et al. A nonsense mutation in COQ9 causes autosomalrecessive neonatal-onset primary coenzyme Q10 deficiency: A potentially treatable form of mitochondrial disease. American Journal of Human Genetics. 2009;**84**:558-566

[36] Lagier-Tourenne C, Tazir M, Lopez LC, Quinzii CM, Assoum M, Drouot N, et al. ADCK3, an ancestral kinase, is mutated in a form of recessive ataxia associated with coenzyme Q10 deficiency. American Journal of Human Genetics. 2008;**82**:661-672

[37] Lopez LC, Schuelke M, Quinzii CM, Kanki T, Rodenburg RJ, Naini A, et al. Leigh syndrome with nephropathy and CoQ10 deficiency due to decaprenyl diphosphate synthase subunit 2 (PDSS2) mutations. American Journal of Human Genetics. 2006;**79**:1125-1129

[38] Mollet J, Delahodde A, Serre V, Chretien D, Schlemmer D, Lombes A, et al. CABC1 gene mutations cause ubiquinone deficiency with cerebellar ataxia and seizures. American Journal of Human Genetics. 2008;**82**:623-630

[39] Mollet J, Giurgea I, Schlemmer D, Dallner G, Chretien D, Delahodde A, et al. Pre-nyldiphosphate synthase, subunit 1 (PDSS1) and OHbenzoate polyprenyltransferase (COQ2) mutations in ubiquinone deficiency and oxidative phosphorylation disorders. The Journal of Clinical Investigation. 2007;**117**:765-772

[40] Quinzii C, Naini A, Salviati L, Trevisson E, Navas P, Dimauro S, et al. A mutation in Para-hydroxybenzoate-polyprenyl transferase (COQ2) causes primary coenzyme Q10 deficiency. American Journal of Human Genetics. 2006;**78**:345-349

[41] Desbats MA, Lunardi G, Doimo M, Trevisson E, Salviati L. Genetic bases and clinical manifestations of coenzyme Q10 (CoQ 10) deficiency. Journal of Inherited Metabolic Disease. 2015;**38**(1):145-156

[42] Quinzii CM, López LC, Naini A, DiMauro S, Hirano M. Human CoQ10 deficiencies. BioFactors. 2008;**32**:113-118

[43] Cobanoglu U, Demir H, Cebi A, Sayir F, Alp HH, Akan Z, et al. Lipid peroxidation, DNA damage and coenzyme Q10 in lung cancer patients–Markers for risk assessment? Asian Pacific Journal of Cancer Prevention. 2011;**12**:1399-1403

[44] Cooper JM, Korlipara LV, Hart PE, Bradley JL, Schapira AH. Coenzyme Q10 and vitamin E deficiency in Friedreich's ataxia: Predictor of efficacy of vitamin E and coenzyme Q10 therapy. European Journal of Neurology. 2008;**15**:1371-1379

[45] Littarru GP, Tiano L. Clinical aspects of coenzyme Q10: An update. Nutrition. 2010;**26**:250-254

[46] Molineux S, Young J, Florkowshi C, Lever M. Coenzyme Q10: Is there a clinical role and a case for measurement? Clinical Biochemist Reviews. 2008;**29**:71-78

[47] Yubero D, Montero R, Martín MA, et al. Secondary coenzyme Q10 deficiencies in oxidative phosphorylation (OXPHOS) and non-OXPHOS disorders. Mitochondrion. 2016;**30**:51-58

[48] Compagnoni G, Lista G, Giuffre B, Mosca F, Marini A. Coenzyme Q10 levels in maternal plasma and cord blood: Correlations with mode of

delivery. Biology of the Neonate. 2004;**86**:104-107

[49] Martinefski MR, Contin MD, Rodriguez MR, Gerez EM, Galleano ML, Lucangioli SE, et al. Coenzyme Q in pregnant women and rats with intrahepatic cholestasis. Liver International. 2014;**34**(7):1040-1048

[50] Martinefski MR, Cocucci SE, Di Carlo MB, Vega HR, Lucangioli SE, Perazzi BE, et al. Fetal coenzyme Q10 deficiency in intrahepatic cholestasis of pregnancy. Clinics and Research in Hepatology and Gastroenterology. 2019;**S2210-7401**(19):30171-30178

[51] Perez MJ, Velasco E, Monte MJ, Gonzalez-BuitragoJM, MarinJJ. Maternal ethanol consumption during pregnancy enhances bile acidinduced oxidative stress and apoptosis in fetal rat liver. Toxicology. 2006a;**225**:183-194

[52] Perez MJ, Macias RI, Duran C, Monte MJ, Gonzalez-Buitrago JM, Marin JJ. Oxidative stress and apoptosis in fetal rat liver induced by maternal cholestasis. Protective effect of ursodeoxycholic acid. Journal of Hepatology. 2005;**43**:324-332

[53] Perez MJ, Macias RI, Marin J. Maternal cholestasis induces placental oxidative stress and apoptosis. Protective effect of ursodeoxycholic acid. Placenta. 2006b;**27**:34-41

[54] Stocker R, Bowry VW. Frei B Ubiquinol-10 protects human low density lipoprotein more efficiently against lipid peroxidation than does alpha-tocopherol. Proceedings of the National Academy of Sciences of the United States of America. 1991;**88**(5):1646-1650

[55] Parola M, Leonarduzzi G, Robino G, Albano E, Poli G, Dianzani MU. On the role of lipid peroxidation in the pathogenesis of liver damage induced by long-standing cholestasis. Free Radical Biology & Medicine. 1996;**20**(3):351-359

[56] Singh S, Shackleton G, Ah-Sing E, Chakraborty J, Bailey ME. Antioxidant defenses in the bile duct-ligated rat. Gastroenterology. 1992;**103**(5):1625-1629

[57] Sokol RJ, Devereaux M, Khandwala RA. Effect of dietary lipid and vitamin E on mitochondrial lipid peroxidation and hepatic injury in the bile duct-ligated rat. Journal of Lipid Research. 1991;**32**(8):1349-1357

[58] Sokol RJ, Winklhofer-Roob BM, Devereaux MW, McKim JM Jr. Generation of hydroperoxides in isolated rat hepatocytes and hepatic mitochondria exposed to hydrophobic bile acids. Gastroenterology. 1995;**109**(4):1249-1256

[59] Aboutwerat A, Pemberton PW, Smith A, Burrows PC, McMahon RF, Jain SK, et al. Oxidant stress is a significant feature of primary biliary cirrhosis. Biochimica et Biophysica Acta. 2003;**1637**(2):142-150

[60] Sokol RJ, Dahl R, Devereaux MW, Yerushalmi B, Kobak GE, Gumpricht E. Human hepatic mitochondria generate reactive oxygen species and undergo the permeability transition in response to hydrophobic bile acids. Journal of Pediatric Gastroenterology and Nutrition. 2005;**41**(2):235-243

[61] Vendemiale G, Grattagliano I, Lupo L, Memeo V, Altomare E. Hepatic oxidative alterations in patients with extra-hepatic cholestasis. Effect of surgical drainage. Journal of Hepatology. 2002;**37**(5):601-605

[62] Krähenbühl S, Talos C, Fischer S, Reichen J. Toxicity of bile acids on the electron transport chain of isolated rat liver mitochondria. Hepatology. 1994;**19**(2):471-479

[63] Yerushalmi B, Dahl R, Devereaux MW, Gumpricht E, Sokol RJ. Bile acid-induced rat hepatocyte apoptosis is inhibited by antioxidants and blockers of the mitochondrial permeability transition. Hepatology. 2001;**33**(3):616-626

[64] Botla R, Spivey JR, Aguilar H, Bronk SF, Gores GJ. Ursodeoxycholate (UDCA) inhibits the mitochondrial membrane permeability transition induced by glycochenodeoxycholate: A mechanism of UDCA cytoprotection. The Journal of Pharmacology and Experimental Therapeutics. 1995;**272**(2):930-938

[65] Dueland S, Reichen J, Everson GT, Davis R. Regulation of cholesterol and bile acid homoeostasis in bile-obstructed rats. The Biochemical Journal. 1991;**280**(Pt 2):373-377

[66] Erickson SK, Jaeckle S, Lear SR, Brady SM, Havel RJ. Regulation of hepatic cholesterol and lipoprotein metabolism in ethinyl estradiol-treated rats. Journal of Lipid Research. 1989;**30**(11):1763-1771

[67] Heuman DM, Hernandez CR, Hylemon PB, Kubaska WM, Hartman C, Vlahcevic ZR. Regulation of bile acid synthesis. I. Effects of conjugated ursodeoxycholate and cholate on bile acid synthesis in chronic bile fistula rat. Hepatology. 1988;**8**(2):358-365

[68] Shefer S, Nguyen L, Salen G, Batta AK, Brooker D, Zaki FG, et al. Feedback regulation of bile-acid synthesis in the rat. Differing effects of taurocholate and tauroursocholate. The Journal of Clinical Investigation. 1990;**85**(4):1191-1198

[69] Davis JM, Auten RL. Maturation of the antioxidant system and the effects on preterm birth. Seminars in Fetal & Neonatal Medicine. 2010;**15**(4): 191-195

[70] Colombo C, Roda A, Roda E, Buscaglia M, dell'gnola CA, Filippetti P, et al. Correlation between fetal and maternal serum bile acid concentrations. Pediatric Research. 1985;**19**(2):227-231

[71] Geenes V, Lövgren-Sandblom A, Benthin L, Lawrance D, Chambers J, Gurung V, et al. The reversed feto-maternal bile acid gradient in intrahepatic cholestasis of pregnancy is corrected by ursodeoxycholic acid. PLoS One. 2014;**9**(1):e83828

[72] Yubero D, Montero R, Armstrong J, Espinós C, Palau F, Santos-Ocaña C, et al. Molecular diagnosis of coenzyme Q10 deficiency. Expert Review of Molecular Diagnostics. 2015;**15**(8):1049-1059